Date: 4/9/19

THE
MOJITO
DIET

THE
MOJITO
DIET

A Doctor-Designed 14-Day
Weight-Loss Plan with a Miami Twist

JUAN RIVERA, MD

ATRIA BOOKS
New York London Toronto Sydney New Delhi

ATRIA
BOOKS

An Imprint of Simon & Schuster, Inc.
1230 Avenue of the Americas
New York, NY 10020

First Atria Books hardcover edition December 2018

ATRIA BOOKS and colophon are trademarks of Simon & Schuster, Inc.

For information about special discounts for bulk purchases,
please contact Simon & Schuster Special Sales at 1-866-506-1949
or business@simonandschuster.com.

The Simon & Schuster Speakers Bureau can bring authors to your
live event. For more information or to book an event, contact the
Simon & Schuster Speakers Bureau at 1-866-248-3049 or visit our
website at www.simonspeakers.com.

Interior design by Jason Snyder

Manufactured in the United States of America

10 9 8 7 6 5 4 3 2 1

Library of Congress Cataloging-in-Publication Data
Names: Rivera, Juan (Juan José), author.
Title: The mojito diet : a doctor-designed 14-day weight loss plan with a
 Miami twist / Juan Rivera, MD.
Description: New York : Atria Books, [2018] | Includes bibliographical
 references and index.
Identifiers: LCCN 2018032979 (print) | LCCN 2018036180 (ebook)
Subjects: LCSH: Reducing diets. | Gluten-free diet. | Fasting. | Weight loss.
Classification: LCC RM222.2 (ebook) | LCC RM222.2 .R555 2018 (print) | DDC
 613.2/5—dc23
LC record available at https://urldefense.proofpoint.com/v2/
url?u=https-3A__lccn.loc.gov_2018032979&d=DwIF-g&c=jGUuvAdBXp_
VqQ6t0yah2g&r=06HB5XcKNe3kUU36TuOk0fMyO_eF5k6L7zVOIl7jYavLVBqUfilIqL
i0uMcjKSVc&m=IvnP2GnjJbXY95u5ZMxWpQ3DRoyG0OAnUc22CAhDIhA&s=j1hj1
MVtPiDLa-3ehxtgubUqzX4XSy6WxdC4K8DGvPs&e=

ISBN 978-1-5011-9201-2
ISBN 978-1-5011-9202-9 (ebook)

I dedicate this book to my wife,
Ana Raquel, and to my children,
Ana Sofia, Juan Antonio, and Nina.

Medical Disclaimer

This book is written for informational purposes only and contains the opinions of the author. It is intended to supplement, but not replace, the advice of your health-care provider. See your doctor or other trained health-care provider before beginning any diet or exercise program, or if you suspect you have a medical condition.

If your doctor has recommended that you take medication for heart disease, high blood pressure, diabetes, or any other medical condition, take it as prescribed.

The weight-loss information in this book is not intended for pregnant or breastfeeding women. See your doctor for advice about the best nutrition and exercise choices during pregnancy and lactation.

Do not drink mojitos or any alcoholic beverage if you have alcoholism, liver disease, or any other medical condition that would be aggravated by alcohol intake; if you are pregnant or may become pregnant; if you take medications that are incompatible with alcohol; or if your doctor has advised you to avoid alcohol for any reason.

CONTENTS

THE
MOJITO
DIET

INTRODUCTION

Lose the Weight, Keep the Fun

A *recent conversation with Sofia*, one of my favorite patients, reminded me of many talks I've had with cardiology patients in the past. Sofia, a forty-nine-year-old hotel executive and the mother of three grown children, has a smile that lights up the room. My staff loves her, and she always begins our appointments by asking me about myself and my family. The world would be a better place with more people like Sofia in it.

Unfortunately, Sofia has several health problems. She takes an ACE inhibitor for high blood pressure and a statin drug for elevated cholesterol. Although she doesn't have type 2 diabetes, her blood sugar is higher than I would like it to be. Sofia's weight had been increasing steadily during the previous few years. During our visit she weighed in at 180 pounds—about 40 pounds over her optimal weight—which for the first time put her into the "obese" category.

Sofia rarely complains, but that day she seemed sad and frustrated. "Lately I've been feeling sluggish and tired," Sofia told me. "I don't seem to have the energy I used to have at work, and trying to keep up with my two-year-old grandson wears me out. My knees have been aching too. I feel like I'm getting old before my time."

Comments like these are very familiar to me. As a board-certified cardiologist and internist who specializes in the prevention, early detection, and treatment of cardiovascular disease, I have many patients whose extra weight interferes with their health, their work, and their ability to enjoy their lives fully. And as the chief medical correspondent for the Univision television network, where I host my own weekly one-hour medical show, *Dr. Juan*, I frequently meet viewers who share their health concerns with me. So many of those who are overweight or obese, like Sofia, worry that symptoms such as shortness of breath, lack of energy, joint pains, and fatigue are warning signs of serious cardiovascular disease. Sometimes they are, but more often they're simply the result of excess weight.

"I'll run some tests to rule out any new medical problems," I assured Sofia during our appointment. "But my guess is that we won't find anything we don't already know about."

"Then why do you think I'm feeling so run-down?"

"Well," I said, glancing at her chart, "you have gained about ten pounds since I last saw you. Carrying around that extra weight could be affecting your energy levels."

Sofia smiled. "I know what you're going to say next. I should go on a diet, right?"

I nodded. Sofia and I had had this conversation before.

"I know it's not easy," I said. "But if you could lose some of those extra pounds, I think you would feel better and more energetic. You'd probably lower your blood sugar. You might even be able to bring down your blood pressure and improve your cholesterol levels. And I bet your knees might even feel better."

"I really would like to lose weight," Sofia explained. "But whenever I look at the diet plans out there, none of them appeal to me." Sofia said she'd heard that high-protein, low-carb diets work well, but she couldn't bear to give up bread, rice, tortillas, and the traditional Cuban comfort foods she'd grown up with. She'd also heard about diets built around a strategy known as intermittent fasting, but she didn't think she could handle the hunger pangs of all-day fasts.

"And alcohol!" Sofia said. "Dr. Juan, don't tell me I can't have a cocktail when I go to a restaurant or a party. We live in Miami, for goodness' sake! You can't ask me to give up my mojitos! I want to lose weight, but I also want to have fun!"

I felt myself break out into a huge smile as I reached for a folder from the stack on my desk. I handed her a copy of my new diet, and her eyes lit up when she read the title.

The Mojito Diet.

"Now *that's* a diet I can follow!"

Weight Loss with a Miami Twist!

I call my weight-loss plan the Mojito Diet not only because the mojito is a popular Miami drink—a favorite of many of my patients, and an excellent reward for weight loss—but because it represents the Latin way of looking at life. The mojito is fresh and bold and effervescent, and so are Latin people. We love to gather with friends and family to celebrate and have fun. Music, dancing, food, and drink are all part of that celebration, as they are for people of many ethnic and cultural backgrounds.

The Mojito Diet makes plenty of room for the bold, flavorful, Latin-inspired foods that people in Miami and across the country associate with fun, festivities, and a hot night out on the town. The recipes in my plan include fantastic dishes that reflect the culinary traditions of Puerto Rico, Mexico, Brazil, Cuba, Spain, and other Latin cuisines, as well as foods that can best be described as Miami fusion—combining a Latin influence with a unique Miami twist. And the Mojito Diet embraces the spirit of celebration with a fitness plan built around traditional Latin dancing and other enjoyable activities that you'll have a blast learning and doing.

The Mojito Diet embraces my philosophy of life—that celebration and joy should be a part of our lives every single day, and that making healthy choices can be a pleasure, not a punishment. Being healthy doesn't have to mean giving up everything you enjoy, or sitting home while everyone else has fun. You can savor life's pleasures in a healthy way. In fact, the best way I can think of to live your life to the fullest is by taking care of your health—and if you're overweight or obese, losing weight is the best place to start celebrating your own life.

A Combination that Works

The Mojito Diet is a fourteen-day plan that succeeds because it combines a high-protein/low-carbohydrate plan, manageable and limited intermittent fasting, and the heart-protective principles of the DASH diet. In short, the Mojito Diet starts where DASH (Dietary Approaches to Stop Hypertension) leaves off: dropping all grains and adding extra protein and fewer carbs during Week 1 (Grain Drop) and three nonconsecutive days of sixteen-hour fasting and adding back healthy amounts of whole grains during Week 2 (Clean 16 Fast). And every week, there are mojitos!

Research has shown us that higher-protein, lower-carbohydrate diets can lead to significant weight loss. But as many people who have tried them have discovered, these diets can be very difficult to stick with for more than a few weeks, because eating so much protein gets very boring. And people following high-protein diets really miss their favorite carbohydrate-rich grain-based foods, such as bread, rice, tortillas, and pasta.

What's more, as a cardiologist, I can't get behind any diet that sidelines the vegetables, fruit, whole grains, nuts, seeds, and legumes that countless studies have associated with cardiovascular health and the potential prevention of a long list of diseases, including dementia and some kinds of cancer. Both the DASH eating plan, which has been shown to lower blood pressure, and the MIND diet (a combination of DASH and the Mediterranean diet), which appears to offer protection from Alzheimer's, include many healthy foods that some low-carbohydrate diets leave off the plate. I can't imagine turning away from foods that have been so strongly associated with good health—that's why you'll find them in the Mojito Diet.

In addition, we have seen that diet plans incorporating certain kinds of fasting can lead to successful weight loss as well as health benefits such as a reduction of inflammation and insulin resistance. However, fasting-based diets can be difficult to follow, because it's hard for people to go for long periods of time without eating. That's why I've created a smart, easy-to-follow sixteen-hour fasting plan—which I refer to as "functional fasting"—that offers the benefits of fasting without the difficulties.

Here's another important roadblock that my eating plan eliminates: I live and practice preventive cardiology in Miami, where people love to party, play, dance, and spend time with family and friends. Asking them to give up the foods and drinks they enjoy, even if doing so may lengthen their lives, is a tough sell. It's especially difficult to convince them to eliminate alcohol—not because they are alcoholics, but because they enjoy drinking alcohol socially. As you can tell from the name of my diet, I don't believe that people have to give up alcohol in order to lose weight—in fact, I think it helps you stay motivated when you think of it as a reward.

When I designed my diet plan, I decided to include the things that *do* work, and to leave out the things that make diets so hard to stick with long-term. The Mojito Diet gives you everything you need for weight-loss success because it focuses on the strategies that work while skipping over the roadblocks that hold you back.

Two Weeks to Forever Weight Loss

Quite simply, my diet plan combines three straightforward strategies that not only produce weight loss and improve heart health but are simple enough that you can do them for the rest of your life.

Week 1

The first half of the Mojito Diet focuses on unleashing the weight-loss properties of protein. As you follow Grain Drop during Week 1 of my fourteen-day diet, you'll avoid all foods that contain grains, such as bread, rice, pasta, and tortillas. Don't worry, you'll still have lots of fantastic foods to eat—I've included dozens of easy recipes for amazingly delicious grain-free breakfasts, lunches, dinners, and snacks. Each day during Grain Drop week, you'll enjoy:

- High-protein foods—such as meat, poultry, seafood, eggs, nuts, legumes, soy, and dairy—at every meal and snack

- Heart-healthy fats
- Plenty of fruits and vegetables throughout the day, with a special emphasis on the high-potassium produce that helps lower blood pressure, such as bananas, sweet potatoes, citrus fruits, spinach, and many others—even white potatoes!

Week 2

During Week 2 of the Mojito Diet, you'll follow my Clean 16 Fast, during which you'll do three nonconsecutive days of sixteen-hour fasts. You will skip breakfast three days of the week (be sure to have your last meal before 8 p.m. the night before). These fasts are easier than they sound, starting after dinner and ending at lunchtime the next day. The Clean 16 Fast is easy to follow, and it has a positive impact on weight loss, insulin resistance, and inflammation. Each day during Clean 16 Fast week, you'll enjoy a wide range of delicious foods, *plus* two to three servings a day of bread, tortillas, or other whole grain foods. Yes! Healthy grains are back.

Until you meet your weight loss goal, you'll alternate following the Week 1 Grain Drop plan and the Week 2 Clean 16 Fast. Then you'll move on to the next phase of the Mojito Diet: the lifetime Mojito Maintenance Plan.

Maintenance

Once you reach your goal weight, you'll shift into my Mojito Maintenance Plan. To maintain your weight loss, you'll follow a healthy eating plan (including grains) five days a week, Grain Drop one day a week, and Clean 16 Fast one day a week. It's that simple.

Plus, Mojitos!

Now, the best part: twice a week during Week 1 and Week 2, and three times a week during Mojito Maintenance, you'll toast your success by rewarding yourself with a refreshing mojito! (Or, if you'd prefer, have another kind of alcoholic beverage or a 200-calorie serving of dessert instead.) Enjoy my favorite Classic Mojito, or choose from among the other delicious mojito recipes included in the book. If you love the refreshing lime-mint taste of mojitos but would rather skip the alcohol, pour yourself a refreshing glass of my Mojito Water (page 198).

The Mojito Diet at a Glance

Week 1: Grain Drop

- No grains! Cut out all breads, rice, pasta, tortillas, and other grains for one week.

- Eat high-protein foods and high-fiber fruits and vegetables at every meal and snack, plus healthy fats.

- Measure your food to learn about healthy portion sizes.

- Reward yourself with two mojitos!

- Drink plenty of water or make my special Mojito Water (page 198).

Week 2: Clean 16 Fast

- Do three nonconsecutive days of sixteen-hour fasts by skipping breakfast three days of the week. (Be sure to finish your last meal before 8 p.m. the night before.)

- On the Clean 16 Fast days, eat a regular lunch and dinner.

- Eat grains again! Have two to three servings of whole grains each day.

- Continue to eat high-protein foods, healthy fats, and high-fiber fruits and vegetables at every meal.

- Don't make up for skipped breakfast by eating more at lunch, snack, or dinner.

- Continue to drink Mojito Water while you fast to fill you up and flush out toxins.

- Reward yourself with two mojitos!

Week 3: Repeat Grain Drop

Week 4: Repeat Clean 16 Fast

After that, continue cycling through the Grain Drop and the Clean 16 Fast, week by week, until you reach your goal weight. Then move on to the Mojito Maintenance Plan.

The Mojito Maintenance Plan

- Eat a healthy diet five days a week.

- Follow the Grain Drop plan one day a week.

- Follow the Clean 16 Fast and skip breakfast one day a week.

- Add extra Grain Drop days if you start to regain lost weight.

- Reward yourself with three mojitos!

Why Weight Loss Matters So Much to Me

If you watch Univision, America's largest Spanish-language television network, you already know me: I'm Univision's chief medical correspondent, and the host of *Dr. Juan*, a weekly one-hour health program. I also co-created and hosted the show *Strange Medicine* and have appeared on other shows on Univision as well as on Telemundo, another Spanish-language network. You may also have seen me in my WebMD video series, *My Abuelita Told Me*, or during my appearances on *Good Morning America*.

I was born and raised in Puerto Rico, where I had an amazing childhood, surrounded by a tight-knit extended family of grandparents, aunts, uncles, and cousins who were like brothers and sisters to me. Working hard in school was the top priority in my family—in my parents' minds, the only question was whether I would become a doctor (as my mother, a social worker, wanted) or an attorney (like my father). When I started medical school at the University of Puerto Rico, I still wasn't quite sure I wanted to be a doctor, and even as I studied classroom-focused subjects such as anatomy and embryology, I questioned my choice. But my interest grew as I started learning about the secrets of the body's physiology, and once I began doing clinical rotations and working directly with patients, I fell in love with medicine. I am a true "people person," and my favorite part of being a doctor is engaging with patients.

I did my residency program in internal medicine at UT Southwestern in Dallas, and was then accepted to the prestigious cardiology fellowship program at The Johns Hopkins Hospital in Baltimore. I started at Johns Hopkins with the goal of becoming an interventional cardiologist. These doctors are the medical superheroes who dramatically save the lives of heart attack victims by performing emergency cardiac catheterizations. As a cardiology fellow, I helped do many of these procedures. During an emergency catheterization, we thread a thin tube into the femoral artery in the patient's leg and guide it through the body to the chest. Using a tiny balloon, we carefully open the blockage in the patient's heart, making it possible for oxygenated blood to flow through the body. Sometimes we implant a stent to keep the blockage from recurring. Performing successful emergency catheterizations is amazing because they can instantaneously save the lives of patients who are just minutes from death. To save a life in this way is an astonishing experience.

However, the excitement I first felt in the cardiac catheterization lab soon disappeared as I realized that I wanted to do more than just rescue heart attack victims from an imminent death. I wanted to help patients earlier—not when they were moments from dying of severe heart disease, but years before that, when they still had time to make lifestyle changes that would protect their hearts and their health long before they suffered heart attacks. I didn't want to *do* catheterizations; I wanted to *prevent* them.

So I decided to become a preventive cardiologist and to shift my focus from heart attack *treatment* to heart disease *prevention* and early detection.

It was a decision that changed the course of my life and helped make me who I am today. And it is the reason I have written this book. I want to show *you* how to lose weight, improve your health, and stay out of the catheterization lab!

I'm a cardiologist and internist with a private concierge practice in Miami Beach. I love my patients, who include business executives, athletes, political leaders, and celebrities from the United States and all over the world. However, when I decided to specialize in heart disease prevention, I also set a very ambitious goal: To help as many people as possible—not just my own patients, but many other people as well.

My number-one value when it comes to medicine is prevention, and having grown up attending Jesuit schools, I am driven by the ideal of service to others. That's why, when I was presented with opportunities to connect with large numbers of people through television and the media, I jumped in with both feet. I love that television allows me to reach so many people—for example, at Univision, I created Reto 28, a twenty-eight-day diet plan that helped four hundred thousand viewers lose more than a million pounds in one month. It was the most successful community initiative in Univision history. My passion is helping people live better, healthier, happier lives.

With my work on television, as well as two bestselling health books and a large social media presence, I've made great progress helping people improve their heart health. Now, with *The Mojito Diet,* I'm hoping to reach even more people, especially the millions of Americans who are overweight or obese.

My message is universal. Heart disease, high blood pressure, and diabetes strike people of all cultures and all backgrounds. These diseases kill more Americans than any others, yet they are surprisingly preventable. Everyone can take simple, important steps—such as losing weight—that can reduce their risk of disease and improve their chances of living a long, healthy life.

One of the best first steps is to start embracing weight loss as an incredible opportunity, rather than a punishing deprivation. You can be happy about being on a diet, because it has the potential to reward you not only with a longer life, but with a greater measure of energy and enjoyment as well. It really is a celebration of life.

By following the Mojito Diet, you can lose weight, improve your health, and have lots of fun along the way. You can eat foods you love, and look forward to rewarding your progress with celebratory mojitos. And count on this: As you set out on your journey to a healthier weight and a better life, I will be with you every step of the way.

PART ONE

CHANGE THE WAY YOU THINK ABOUT WEIGHT LOSS

To lose weight, you can't just change the way you eat or how much you move. You also have to change the way you *think*.

You're more likely to shed pounds and keep them off for good if you think of diet and exercise as amazing opportunities to feel better and to be healthier, rather than as punishments you must endure in order to squeeze into smaller-size clothing. In part 1 of this book, I'll show you how to do that.

In this section, we'll look at ways to shift the way you think about food, activity, and weight loss. We'll explore some of the incredible health benefits that can start coming your way within days of starting the Mojito Diet. And I'll give you some very specific strategies for shifting your weight-loss mind-set and using rewards to bring about success.

I'll also share some great ideas about how to change the way you think about fitness. If you haven't enjoyed exercise in the past, get ready to start loving it!

The Mojito Diet looks at diet and exercise in an entirely new way. It doesn't have to be a bore or a chore. I want you to have fun while losing weight!

1

Why Bother to Lose Weight?

I want to start this book by telling you something very important: You don't have to be thin to be sexy.

I live in Miami, which prides itself on being a sexy city full of attractive people, a warm place with cool beaches and a hot nightlife. People in Miami embrace this sensual ambience. You can see it in the way they dress, the way they dance, the way they move even when they're just walking down the street or out doing errands. You should see them at Miami Heat games—it's like being at a fashion show! Miami fans dress as if they, rather than the basketball players, are the stars of the show. I admit to being slightly biased on this topic, but I think Miamians are some of the most gorgeous people in the world, whatever their size. Their beauty comes from their sense of confidence, style, and playfulness, their friendliness and kindness, and their openhearted way of presenting themselves to the world, embracing the pleasures of life, and refusing to take themselves too seriously.

From the standpoint of appearances, I don't care what size you are. You can be beautiful, confident, and sexy at any weight. You can be an amazing spouse, parent, friend, neighbor, or employee no matter what your shape. If it were only about the number on the scale or the size of your clothing, I'd tell you not to worry at all about what you weigh, because beauty comes in all shapes and sizes.

But, unfortunately, weight isn't just about numbers. Weight and health are intricately linked. Although it is possible for overweight or obese people to be healthy, you're much more likely to experience a long list of health problems if you carry excess weight, and you're much more likely to be in better health if you're closer to a normal weight. You can absolutely be beautiful if you weigh too much—but you may not be very healthy.

That's why, if you are overweight or obese, I want you to try to lose weight.

I know—it's not easy. You've probably tried to lose weight before. Perhaps you've attempted it many times. Maybe you've succeeded, but gained the weight back. Or maybe this is the first time you'll be doing it. Your history doesn't matter—what does matter is that you've picked up this book. You're willing to give weight loss a try. You're ready to start following an eating and activity plan that will bring you closer to good health.

I cannot tell you how proud I am of you for taking this step.

Weight loss is hard—if it were simple, there wouldn't be so many overweight and obese people, and diet books wouldn't be so popular. But even though it's not easy, it is doable. It's possible to lose excess pounds and move yourself into a healthier place. You can do it.

The people who succeed at losing weight and keeping it off have a few things in common. They follow a diet plan that includes the healthy foods their bodies need as well as many of their favorite meals—a diet plan that boosts their enjoyment of food while reducing the amount of food (and the amount of unhealthy food) they eat. Successful weight losers also figure out a way to make physical activity a pleasurable part of their everyday lives. They don't force themselves to do workouts they don't like. Rather, they identify activities they love and work them into their schedules in a way that brings them happiness and satisfaction. And they reward themselves for their hard work. Personally, I have tried many different physical activities throughout my life, including weight lifting, marathon running, boxing, insanity workouts, and Pilates. I am constantly changing the activities I do without fear of trying new ones—although I've learned (the hard way) not to take it too seriously, as I did when I took up boxing and broke my wrist and a rib while sparring. Now I just punch bags, because they don't hit back!

Five Reasons to Lose Weight

As you follow the Mojito Diet, you'll eat foods you love, engage in activities you enjoy, and move yourself closer to a healthy weight. But before we start going into detail about the various elements of the Mojito Diet, I think it's important for us to talk about the health-related reasons to commit yourself to weight loss. If you don't truly believe that weight loss is important, you'll be less likely to succeed. Understanding and embracing the health benefits of weight loss can make it easier for you to stay committed to your goals.

As I mentioned earlier, I don't want you to lose weight for the sake of your looks, because I think people of all shapes and sizes can be sexy and beautiful. I want you to drop those extra pounds so you can be healthier—so you can live longer, have a stronger heart, have the stamina to do the activities you enjoy, and maybe even take less medication. When you're making the choices you must make to lose weight—choices that are sometimes challenging or difficult—I want you to be able to think about the benefits you'll be bringing to your health.

I've seen people try to lose weight to fit into the jeans they wore in high school or the bikini they wore on their honeymoon. Those are fun goals to have, but from what I've seen with my patients, they're just not compelling enough to keep you from eating a big piece of cake or having a second serving of chiles rellenos. Thinking about the ways in which saying "no, thank you" to cake or second servings will benefit your health is, in my experience, a much more powerful motivator.

And so, in this chapter, let's look at the answers to the question of why you should even bother to lose weight, improve your diet, and become more active. It's about your health, not your looks. Understanding the *why* of weight loss can go a long way toward motivating you to long-term success, helping you lose those extra pounds, and reducing your risk of many of our most common causes of death and disability.

Reason #1: A Lower Risk of Heart Disease

Hey, I'm a cardiologist, so of course I'm going to start by talking about heart health. What else would you expect of me?

Your heart is a muscle that pumps blood throughout your body. It really is an amazing organ—it starts to beat before you are born and continues working nonstop until death. It never takes a break. If you're lucky enough to live to the age of, say, eighty, your heart will have beaten more than three billion times. When your heart beats, blood flows into your heart and then travels to your lungs, where it picks up oxygen and drops off carbon dioxide. The oxygenated blood then travels through your body, where blood vessels deliver it to organs, tissues, and cells. When your heart stops beating, death occurs within minutes.

Unfortunately, many people develop various kinds of heart and blood vessel diseases, which are referred to as cardiovascular disease or simply heart disease. Heart disease is a massive health problem in the United States and around the world. It is the number-one cause of death in the United States, killing more than eight hundred thousand people every year. It also causes enormous pain and suffering for patients and their families.

There are many factors that influence whether you'll get heart disease, and, if you do have it, whether it will lead to an early death. For example, certain genetic factors play a part in heart disease. But overall, the risk of developing most kinds of heart disease is heavily influenced by the lifestyle choices we make every day—whether we smoke, how much we eat, what kinds of foods we eat, whether we are active, and whether we take steps to prevent or manage high blood pressure, control cholesterol, and reduce high blood sugar.

To me, the biggest tragedy of heart disease is how preventable it is. Studies have found that at least half of all heart disease deaths could be prevented. Half! And what's even more incredible is that the ways in which heart disease can be prevented are quite simple—not through major medical interventions, but with straightforward changes in how people live their daily lives, such as losing weight, exercising, and not smoking. Think about that for a minute: Just by making different choices on a day-to-day basis, we could prevent as many as four hundred thousand premature deaths in the United States *every year.* Imagine it! We could save the lives of four hundred thousand husbands, wives, parents, siblings, grandparents, and friends each year with simple lifestyle choices like the ones in this book.

Reason #2: Better Blood Pressure

Getting your blood pressure to a better place is another reason to lose weight if you are overweight or obese. Having high blood pressure, also known as hypertension, is not good because it raises your risk of heart disease and stroke, two of the top causes of death in the United States. About seventy-five million adults in this country—about one in three—have high blood pressure. An additional seventy-five million Americans have prehypertension, which means their blood pressure is higher than it should be, but not high enough to receive a diagnosis of high blood pressure—yet.

Here's what it means to have high blood pressure: When your heart pumps, blood travels through your blood vessels throughout your body. Blood pressure is the force that your blood exerts against the walls of your blood vessels. If that force is too high, you have a condition that we refer to as hypertension, or high blood pressure.

You can help bring down your blood pressure by making some important changes: quitting smoking, cutting back on or eliminating alcohol if you drink too much, eating a healthier diet (such as the Mojito Diet) that includes less sodium and more potassium, being more active, and losing weight. Your doctor may recommend that you take blood pressure medication; if so, be sure to take it as prescribed.

Because high blood pressure is such a prevalent problem, I have designed the Mojito Diet with prevention very much in mind. We'll talk about this more in chapter 9, but for now, it's important for you to know that many of the nutritional recommendations in the Mojito Diet are based on what we've learned from the science behind the DASH (Dietary Approaches to Stop Hypertension) eating plan. By following my eating plan, you can lose weight and lower your blood pressure at the same time.

Reason #3: Lower Blood Sugar

The third very important reason for you to lose weight if you are overweight or obese is that doing so can help improve your blood sugar levels and lower your risk of developing type 2 diabetes or prediabetes.

Type 2 diabetes is a serious disease. It is also quite prevalent: More than thirty million Americans have it—that's about 10 percent of the overall population. In Americans over age sixty-five, about 25 percent have type 2 diabetes. It used to be thought of as a disease of old age, but as the obesity epidemic has grown, alarming numbers of younger adults, teens, and even children now develop it.

There are other kinds of diabetes, such as type 1 diabetes and gestational diabetes, which occurs during pregnancy. But I want to focus here on type 2 diabetes because it's the most common, and it is the version of the disease that is most closely linked with excess weight. In fact, 80 percent of people who have diabetes are either overweight or obese.

Type 2 diabetes is something I think about often, because it runs in my family. Both of my parents have diabetes—in fact, I diagnosed my own mother earlier in my career. She came into my new cardiology office, so proud of her son, so thrilled to have me giving her a checkup. But when I ran an HbA1c test that measures average blood sugar levels for the previous few months, I discovered that hers was 12.3 percent, which was much higher than the optimal measure of 5.7 percent.

Unfortunately, I also tend to have high blood sugar, which is one of the reasons exercise and a healthy diet are so important to me. I'm pretty good about eating well, but I must admit, I have a sweet tooth. You might even call me a sugar addict, although in the past five or six years I've taken control of my sugar addiction. Years ago, sugar had a big hold on me. If I went out to dinner, I'd choose the restaurant based on its dessert menu! When I was a cardiology fellow at Johns Hopkins, I lived three blocks away from a fantastic ice cream parlor, and I had ice cream almost every day. Now I eat it maybe once a year. I want to keep my blood sugar in a healthy place.

That emphasis on sugar is a hallmark of Hispanic culture. When I grew up in Puerto Rico, my family would have dessert every evening—often several choices, in fact. My father wouldn't get up from the dinner table unless a dessert had been served. Many of the favorite foods in Latin cuisine are carbohydrate-heavy, which is also not good for blood sugar. Now I am hyperaware of sugar in foods, and I avoid it whenever possible—I only have dessert on special occasions, and I have cut back on my overall carbohydrate intake by reducing the bread, rice, and other grains in my diet. I check my own HbA1c regularly; if I am not conscientious about my eating and exercise, my blood sugar starts to creep up into the prediabetes range. I even continue to exercise while on vacation, because if I don't, I'm likely to gain five pounds or so from all those restaurant meals. For me, even a five-pound weight gain is enough to increase my blood sugar significantly. Luckily, I enjoy exercise, which has a very positive effect on blood sugar, as we'll discuss in chapter 4.

In people with type 2 diabetes, blood glucose (blood sugar) levels get too high. Here's how that happens: When you eat food, your body breaks it down in order to use it. Insulin, a hormone that's made by your pancreas, moves the glucose in foods from your blood into your cells, where they use it for energy. If your pancreas doesn't make enough insulin—which is what happens in people with diabetes—or if your body doesn't use insulin properly, glucose stays in your blood instead of moving into your cells. People who are overweight or obese can become resistant to insulin, which means their cells have trouble taking in blood sugar, allowing too much of it to stay in their blood.

Having too much glucose in your blood can cause damage to many parts of your body, including your heart, blood vessels, nerves, kidneys, eyes, feet, and sexual organs. Nerve damage from diabetes, which is known as diabetic neuropathy, is serious business: It can cause pain, dizziness, weakness, gastrointestinal difficulties, sexual dysfunction, and other health problems. Sadly, it can also lead to foot or limb amputation in extreme cases.

You may be at risk even if you're not one of the more than thirty million people in the United States who have type 2 diabetes. A huge number of people—eighty-four million Americans, or one in three people—have a condition called prediabetes (also known as impaired glucose tolerance, impaired fasting glucose, or borderline diabetes). With prediabetes, your blood sugar is higher than it should be, but not quite high enough to be considered diabetes. If you have prediabetes, there's a good chance that, unless you make some important changes in your life, you'll develop type 2 diabetes within a few years. Having prediabetes also raises your risk of heart disease.

So that's the bad news about type 2 diabetes.

The good news is that if you have type 2 diabetes or prediabetes, or if you are at risk for developing them, you can take three important steps to lower your blood sugar and improve your health: losing weight, becoming more active, and eating a healthier diet.

Studies have found that weight loss brought about by eating healthy foods and exercising can have a pretty amazing impact on your likelihood of developing type 2 diabetes. In fact, a large study known as the Diabetes Prevention Program (DPP), which looked at behavior changes in people with prediabetes, found that losing weight through diet and exercise lowered the risk of developing diabetes by 58 percent. This is an incredible discovery! And what's equally exciting is that the study found that even small amounts of weight reduction can have an impact—losing just 5 to 7 percent of your body weight can lower the risk of developing type 2 diabetes. In other words, if you weigh two hundred pounds, you can make a difference by losing just ten to fourteen pounds. When people with type 2 diabetes lose weight, they can often reduce their need for diabetes medications. Some studies have even suggested that type 2 diabetes may actually be reversible with weight loss. Here's another remarkable finding from the DPP study: Weight loss and exercise did a better job of preventing type 2 diabetes than taking the diabetes drug metformin. That's right. Lifestyle changes like the ones I recommend in the Mojito Diet were more effective at lowering type 2 diabetes risk than a diabetes drug. If that doesn't convince you that losing weight and becoming more active offer protection from type 2 diabetes, I don't know what will.

Weight loss and exercise help your body use insulin more effectively. Not only does this help lower your blood sugar, but it can also reduce blood pressure, improve your cholesterol levels, and have a positive impact on other diabetes risk factors. It's definitely a win-win situation.

If you are at risk for type 2 diabetes, or if you have prediabetes, you don't just have to sit back and accept it. You can take charge of your health and lower your risk by improving your diet, becoming more active, and losing weight. You can do all of those things simply by following the Mojito Diet.

Reason #4: A Reduced Risk of Cancer

After heart disease, cancer is the number-two cause of death in the United States. Not all kinds of cancer are linked to excess weight, but some are, including postmenopausal breast cancer and cancers of the colon and rectum (referred to as colorectal cancer), endometrium (the lining of the uterus), esophagus, stomach, liver, pancreas, gallbladder, and kidney.

Researchers don't fully understand why cancer risk goes up in people who are overweight or obese. They believe that fat cells may release hormones that help cancer cells grow; the more fat cells a person has, the more cancer-feeding hormones are released, according to that theory. Researchers also know that obese people tend to have higher levels of chronic inflammation throughout their bodies, which can damage cells over time. Also, there's evidence that eating a diet that contains lots of processed foods and low levels of healthy foods such as fruits and vegetables is associated with certain kinds of cancers.

If you're concerned about getting cancer—and really, who wouldn't be?—you're in good hands with the Mojito Diet. While following my eating plan, you'll have plenty of the kinds of foods that help lower the risk of some types of cancer. Take colorectal cancer, for example. Lots of studies have found that eating a high-fiber diet that includes a rainbow of fruits and vegetables—like the Mojito Diet—can help lower the risk of colorectal cancer. Losing weight offers colorectal cancer protection too, as do eating nuts, healthy fats, and fatty fish such as salmon; replacing processed white breads and grains with whole grains; and cutting back on red meats.

Reason #5: Better Overall Health

Losing weight can significantly lower the risk of heart disease, high blood pressure, type 2 diabetes, and cancer, our biggest causes of death and disability. But there are many other health-related reasons to lose weight. If you're overweight or obese, shedding some of those extra pounds can benefit nearly every system in your body.

For example, if you have joint pain, losing weight could help reduce that pain by taking some of the pressure off your joints. If you have trouble getting a good night's sleep because of obstructive sleep apnea, weight loss could lead to a better night's rest. And if your weight interferes with your sexual performance, dropping some extra pounds could allow you to have more fun in bed. The list of benefits really is almost endless. Some of the many other health conditions that may improve with weight loss include asthma, back pain, chronic kidney disease, dementia risk, depression, gallstones and gallbladder disease, gastrointestinal problems, gout, infertility, insomnia, joint pain, leg and foot pain, low energy, nonalcoholic fatty liver disease, and osteoarthritis, as well as pregnancy complications such as gestational diabetes, preeclampsia, the need for cesarean delivery, preterm birth, and neural tube defects in the baby's brain and spinal cord.

DR. JUAN'S WISDOM

STAND UP TO YOUR FAMILY HEALTH HISTORY

High blood pressure often runs in families and seems to have a genetic component. However, as I often tell my patients, just because you have high blood pressure in your family doesn't mean you are destined to get it. You have more power over hypertension than you realize.

You can help prevent high blood pressure—or help lower it, if it's already elevated—with lifestyle changes such as weight loss, exercise, eating better, quitting smoking, and cutting back on alcohol if you drink excessively. I've seen patients bring their blood pressure down significantly by making these changes in their lives; some even reduce or eliminate their need for blood pressure medication.

A New Weight-Loss Mind-Set

I want you to keep all of these health benefits in mind as you get started on the Mojito Diet. You have so much to gain from losing weight. But listen—I know that simply being aware of the health advantages of weight loss isn't necessarily enough to motivate you to change your diet and become more active. Sadly, I've watched people who have continued to smoke, be inactive, or eat unhealthy foods after suffering a heart attack. It is astonishing, but quite true. You'd think a heart attack would provide the motivation necessary to lose weight or make other important lifestyle changes, but for some people, even a brush with death doesn't offer enough incentive.

By watching and learning from the people who do succeed at making crucial health changes, I've discovered an important lesson: To achieve important health behavior changes such as long-term weight loss, you don't just have to alter what you eat or how you move. You have to transform the way you think—about food, about activity, and about your overall health. Changing your thought patterns is as important as changing your eating and exercise patterns.

Adjusting the way you think might sound hard, but it is actually simpler than you may realize. In fact, psychologists have come up with some ingenious ways to help people learn how to restructure the negative thought patterns that may interfere with achieving their important life goals, such as losing weight. That's why, in the next chapter, I'm going to introduce you to some new ways to think about weight loss, healthy eating, and activity, as well as some important suggestions for getting past your emotional roadblocks. Using these strategies, you can begin to change some of the thinking habits that may have prevented you from losing weight in the past, and develop thought patterns that can help pave the way for your future weight-loss success.

MOJITO DIET SUCCESS STORY: **LESLIE**

Losing Weight After Childbirth

Leslie wanted to drop some extra weight after having her third child. Even though she was working out, the baby weight just wouldn't come off. "I needed to get back in shape," says Leslie, forty, a journalist and chief editor of a magazine. "I was exercising about four times a week, but exercise was not enough."

When I mentioned the Mojito Diet to Leslie, she was reluctant to give it a try. "I'm not the type of girl who is obsessed with her weight. And for me to do a diet is a very big deal because I'm a foodie!" But Leslie took a look at the Mojito Diet and decided to give it a chance because it made sense to her.

Leslie started losing weight right away. And she experienced other changes as well. "I was bloated all the time, and that is so much better now," Leslie says. Within six weeks, Leslie had lost nine pounds and two inches off her waist.

"I fit so much better into my clothes now—I don't have a belly going over my jeans!" Leslie says. "And also, I don't suffer from the heat as much—not to mention how my husband looks at me differently."

Leslie liked that the Mojito Diet wasn't "painful" for her to follow, and that she didn't feel like she had to restrain herself. "I was eating, and I never felt hungry for a minute," she says. "I am so happy that I had the chance to try this diet because it has changed my silhouette and shape already. And it is so easy that I am simply not stopping the diet!"

2

~~~~~

Change Your
Weight-Loss Mind-Set

I saw so much regret during my cardiology medical training.

As a cardiac fellow at Johns Hopkins, I worked with many heart attack patients. Often they were rushed to the hospital with crushing chest pain caused by blockages in their hearts. My fellow physicians and I performed emergency catheterizations in the hopes of opening their blocked hearts to allow blood to flow freely again. The lucky patients survived, but some did not. The damage to their hearts was simply too severe, and there was nothing we could do to save them.

When I'd check on these heart attack patients after their procedures, they often told me stories of great despair. They sorely regretted the choices that may have contributed to their heart attacks. I would be a very wealthy man if I had received a dollar every time one of those patients said, "I should have quit smoking years ago!" or "I should have exercised more!" or "I should have lost weight."

Regret is a painful emotion that can cause immense guilt and shame. When you're lying in a hospital bed after having suffered a heart attack, you can't go back into the past and change your actions. Cardiac rehabilitation programs can do wonders for patients who are willing to work on improving their health, but nothing can erase a heart attack.

Heart patients' stories of regret were one of the reasons I decided to become a preventive cardiologist—and write this book. I wanted to show people how to make changes that would help them avoid heart attacks, stay out of the hospital, and bypass the devastating feelings of regret that plague heart attack victims. In my experience, the feelings of regret that many heart patients feel are often more painful to them than their heart attacks.

And so, with the memories of those patients in my mind, I am determined to help you avoid their fate.

Going Beyond Goals

Here's an important lesson I have learned. Just telling people what they should or shouldn't do usually isn't enough. Most of the heart attack patients who expressed so much regret while lying in the intensive care unit after their emergency procedures knew what they should have done to avoid heart disease. But they didn't do it. They didn't quit smoking or lose weight or eat healthier foods or start exercising.

For many of them, part of the problem was that although they knew what they should do — such as losing weight — they didn't know exactly how to do it. They might have had a goal, but not a plan. For example, one woman I spoke to said she didn't exercise because the one time she tried to go for a run, she got so winded that she never tried it again. Unfortunately, she didn't realize that walking would have been a better activity for her anyway.

Another patient told me he would have liked to lose weight, but he felt that cutting back on the traditional foods his wife cooked would have been an insult to her. I could relate to that story. My grandmother was an excellent cook. Her food was out-of-this-world delicious! But to make her happy and show your appreciation for her cooking, you had to eat everything on your plate and go for seconds. That would bring a smile to my *abuela's* face, but it also meant a lot of food (and calories) in our bellies.

Part of the solution to these challenges is choosing a weight-loss plan like the Mojito Diet that makes room for foods you like in a healthy diet and that guides you to choose fitness activities you enjoy, such as dancing or doing fun-walks with friends. But there's more to it than that.

To boost your chances of losing weight and keeping it off forever, you have to do more than just make adjustments to your diet and activity levels.

You have to change the way you think.

Your outlook really does matter. I've seen it many times with my patients: The ones who are most successful at losing weight are the ones who have what I think of as a positive weight-loss mind-set, rather than a negative weight-loss mind-set.

There's no doubt in my mind that negative thinking about weight loss holds people back, and positive thinking propels them forward. That's why I'm going to help you reframe your negative thoughts so that you can think about diet, activity, and weight loss in a more positive, constructive, optimistic way.

Instead of thinking of a weight-loss plan as a grueling punishment, I want you to think of it as an amazing opportunity to feel better and improve your health.

Instead of thinking of eating a healthy diet as an annoying deprivation, I want you to think of it as an exciting chance to experiment with new foods and flavors, and to rediscover how delicious food can be without lots of added salt and sugar.

Instead of thinking of exercise as a horrible chore, I want you to think of it as a pleasurable way to energize your body, socialize with friends, and feel younger than you have in years.

Instead of dreading the start of this diet, I want you to feel excited about it!

All right, all right. I know what you're probably thinking: "Dr. Juan, this all sounds good. But *how* am I supposed to change the way I think about diets, exercise, and weight loss?" That's what we're going to discuss in this chapter.

Building a More Helpful Mind-Set

Psychologists have learned quite a lot lately about how to help people reframe their negative self-talk in ways that help them look at things in a more beneficial way. They've identified a three-step process that you can use to identify and restructure the negative thoughts that interfere with your ability to meet your goals.

In other words, by adjusting your mind-set, you can make it easier for yourself to succeed at weight loss (or whatever other goals you have). That's true because our thoughts can have a big impact on our choices, and our choices can have a big impact on our health. By changing your thoughts, you can change your actions. By having a more positive outlook about eating, activity, and weight loss, you can make better choices that will benefit your weight and your health.

It comes down to this: If you think of a weight-loss plan as a punishment, you're less likely to succeed. But if you can shift your outlook and think of it as an incredible opportunity that you're lucky to have, you'll be well on your way to victory.

Changing your weight-loss mind-set is easier if you follow this three-step plan.

Step 1: Identify your automatic negative thoughts about healthy eating, exercise, and weight loss

Automatic thoughts are the ones that pop up in your mind in an unconscious, reactive way. Most of us aren't aware of our automatic thoughts—they're so familiar to us that we accept them as fact and don't think to question them. We think of them as truth, rather than opinion. Our automatic thoughts can be influenced by many things, including our family, friends, cultural values, life experiences, religious background, education, and the media.

It's good to become aware of your automatic thoughts because they can have a great deal of power over you. Automatic thoughts can trigger feelings that inspire you (such as happiness, enthusiasm, excitement) or challenge you (stress, anxiety, sadness, anger, self-loathing). They can also affect your actions and guide your decisions. Although in this book you and I are talking about those related to diet, exercise, and weight loss, our unconscious reactions and automatic thoughts affect every part of our lives, from our relationships to our careers.

Unfortunately, our automatic thoughts aren't always helpful to us. Often they're not even accurate, and they may be quite negative and destructive. This stream of negative self-talk can be like a radio station playing in the back of your mind, repeating hurtful thoughts over and over and over. Negative automatic thoughts can do great harm if they interfere with your ability to take care of yourself and make healthy choices. In some cases, they can even contribute to mental health conditions such as depression and anxiety.

Here's an example of negative self-talk that is common among people who are overweight or obese. When they get on the scale and see that their weight has gone up, their first thought is, "What a pig I am!" or "I am such a failure!" We would never talk to our friends or family in this way, yet we say things like this to ourselves all the time.

We aren't stuck with our automatic negative thoughts. We can take control of them and restructure them in a way that helps take away their harmful power. But before we can restructure them, we must identify them.

The best way to do this is to spend some time listening to yourself think. Pay close attention to your self-talk and your automatic thoughts when you do anything related to your weight—eating, exercising, weighing yourself, even reading this book. Anytime you notice an automatic negative thought, jot it down in a journal, a notebook, or a document file on your phone or computer. Keeping a record of your automatic negative thoughts is important because we're going to come back to them in the next two steps.

As you set out to identify your automatic negative thoughts, be on the lookout for the following thinking patterns:

All-or-nothing thinking: Judging yourself or your actions as being completely effective or completely useless. You may be engaging in all-or-nothing thinking (also known as black-and-white thinking) if you believe that unless you can lose *all* your excess weight, there's no point in even trying to lose *some* weight.

Perfectionism: Believing that if you don't do something 100 percent perfectly, you are a total failure. This comes up all the time in people who are trying to lose weight. They start a diet or an exercise program, expect themselves to follow it perfectly, and then declare themselves or their plans a failure when they slip up and eat one cookie or fail to lose a large amount of weight in a short amount of time. Rather than accepting that they made a mistake and keep trying, they give up.

Filtering: Seeing only negatives and ignoring positives. For example, you may engage in filtering if you lie in bed at night dwelling on the one poor eating choice you made that day rather than feeling proud of the many healthy choices you made.

Fallacy of fairness: Expecting life to be fair and feeling annoyed and angry when it isn't. You know what this is if you feel unreasonably upset when you spend time with a thin friend who can eat whatever she wants and not gain a pound. No, it's not fair that you have a weight problem and she doesn't. But life isn't always fair.

Negative forecasting: Making pessimistic assumptions about future outcomes. Examples of this include "I'll never be able to lose weight" and "There's no point in trying to learn salsa dancing because I won't be able to do it well." When we engage in negative forecasting, we allow the worst possible outcomes of an action to influence us as we make decisions.

Emotional decision-making: Allowing emotions to affect your choices. Perhaps you decide to eat a chocolate bar because you are sad, or decide not to exercise because you're upset about something that happened at work. You may think you can't improve your diet because you "hate" healthy foods, or you "can't stand" to exercise.

"Should" or "must" thinking: Believing the "should" or "must" statements that pop into your mind, such as "I should have better self-control," or "I should not be overweight," or "I must eat everything on my plate." These kinds of statements can prevent you from taking care of yourself because they can lead you to feel overwhelmed by unrealistic expectations.

Comparison to others: Judging yourself and your actions in comparison to other people, usually in a very unrealistic way that leaves you feeling inferior and ashamed. How many times have you compared yourself to thinner friends and family members? Think of how that makes you feel. Pay attention to the comments that others make to you too. Even well-meaning remarks can interfere with your success.

Overgeneralizing: Making generalizations without adequate evidence. This often happens when people try new things—one of my patients gave in to overgeneralization when she tried taking a Zumba class at her gym. She felt awkward during the first few minutes of class. Even though the instructor assured the participants that it was completely normal to feel awkward when starting Zumba, my patient threw in the towel after about ten minutes and gave up on the class. Lucky for her, she reconsidered her overgeneralization, gave Zumba another try, and soon fell in love with it.

As you consider the automatic negative thoughts that pop into your head when you think about healthy eating, exercise, and weight loss, be sure to write them down. Once you've got a list, you're ready to move on to the next step.

Step 2: Challenge your automatic negative thoughts

During this step, I'd like you to look at each of the automatic negative thoughts that you've written down and challenge them. Because our automatic thoughts are so familiar to us—many of them have been rattling around in our heads since childhood or young adulthood—we take them at face value and believe them as truth. But they're often very inaccurate. Even if they contain a grain of truth, that grain is usually wrapped in layers of exaggeration and overstatement.

Challenging automatic negative thoughts means putting them to the test and analyzing them to determine whether they are true. You can challenge your thoughts using some of the following questions:

- Is this thought accurate?

- What is the evidence to support this thought?

- Am I oversimplifying my view of the situation?

- Why do I think this? Is it something that I grew up hearing without ever stopping to think about whether it was accurate?

- Is this thought based on feelings rather than facts?

- Am I overemphasizing the negative aspect of the situation and downplaying the positive?

- If this thought does include a kernel of truth, is there a way to think about it that acknowledges the truth but removes layers of exaggeration and overstatement?

- Is it harmful for me to believe this thought?

I think you'll discover that as you challenge your negative self-talk, many of the automatic thoughts that flow through your mind on a regular basis are much less accurate than you might have expected.

Now that you've put some of your negative thoughts to the test, you're ready to move on to the final step.

Step 3: Restructure your automatic negative thoughts

This is the most satisfying step of the process because it allows you an opportunity to talk back to your automatic negative thoughts and restructure them in a way that is more accurate, more helpful to you, and less likely to cause you stress. When you restructure negative thoughts, you create more positive, balanced ways of looking at a situation. Your revised thought can be more accurate, optimistic, and helpful to you than the automatic negative thought. By restructuring your negative self-talk, you have the power to change hurtful thoughts into helpful thoughts.

Here are some examples of how you can redirect your negative self-talk.

▶ HURTFUL NEGATIVE THOUGHT: I am such a loser for allowing myself to gain all this weight in the first place.

Helpful restructured thought: I am being way too hard on myself here. Other than a small number of people who are naturally thin—the ones who can eat anything and not gain an ounce—most of us struggle with weight. I am not a loser or a failure or a disappointment. I am a good person who happens to be facing the same challenge that two-thirds of all Americans face. I am also a strong person, so if I want to lose weight, I can do it. But there is nothing wrong with me as a human being because I carry some extra pounds. I am a valuable person no matter what I weigh.

▸ **HURTFUL NEGATIVE THOUGHT:** Having to lose weight is a punishment, and I'm angry about having to do it.

Helpful restructured thought: It's true, there are things about embarking on a weight-loss plan that are bothersome and inconvenient. I don't like the idea of having to pay attention to what I eat or how much I eat, and I would rather not have to exercise. But I have a choice here. I can make these changes and improve my health, or I can just keep going as in the past, eating too much and avoiding activity. Unfortunately, if I don't make any changes, I won't feel any better, and my risk of serious heart disease and other health problems will continue to go up. As the saying goes, nothing changes if nothing changes. However, if I do try to eat a healthier diet and start being more active, it's likely that I'll begin to feel better and lower my health risks. I may feel more energetic and sleep better, and my mood may improve, as is the case with many people who lose weight. I wish I didn't have to go on a diet—no, it's not fair that I have a weight problem and other people don't. But I've been given many blessings that other people haven't. We all have our burdens and our challenges, and weight loss happens to be my challenge right now. I'm going to try to let go of my anger and face this challenge with a positive attitude and think of it as an opportunity rather than a punishment.

▸ **HURTFUL NEGATIVE THOUGHT:** I'm not going to bother exercising for only ten minutes. If I can't work out for an hour, there's no point in exercising at all.

Helpful restructured thought: It's true, an hour of exercise is better than ten minutes. But ten minutes of activity is much better than nothing at all, and if I wait until I have a full hour to exercise, I may not get around to it for days. Dr. Juan said that intermittent bursts of activity throughout the day are as useful as longer workouts, so if I have ten minutes, I'm going to take advantage of it and get moving right away!

▶ **HURTFUL NEGATIVE THOUGHT**: If I can't lose all my extra weight and get back to what I weighed in high school, I'm not going to bother losing any weight at all.

Helpful restructured thought: Yes, it would be wonderful to be as slim as I was when I was eighteen. But it's actually a very unrealistic goal, because it's been years since my weight was that low—and I've had three children since then! Expecting to lose that much weight is preventing me from trying to drop any weight at all. I am going to set a more realistic goal for now. When I get there, I'll consider setting another goal for the future.

▶ **HURTFUL NEGATIVE THOUGHT**: It's impossible for me to lose enough weight to improve my health.

Helpful restructured thought: This is completely untrue. In chapter 1, Dr. Juan discussed a study that found that a loss of as little as 5 to 7 percent of a person's body weight can result in a reduced risk of type 2 diabetes and other health problems. Losing 5 to 7 percent of my weight is a very realistic goal. Sure, if I can lose more than that, my health risks could decrease even more. But starting with a 5 percent weight loss is an excellent first step that will not only be good for my health, but will most likely make me feel better also.

▶ **HURTFUL NEGATIVE THOUGHT**: I will be miserable if I go on a diet because I won't be able to live without my favorite desserts and my usual two glasses of wine each evening.

Helpful restructured thought: It's true that if I change my diet and start to eat healthier foods, I'll have to make some sacrifices. For example, I'll have to cut back on ice cream and brownies, two of my favorite foods. And all that wine isn't helpful for my weight or my overall health. But with the Mojito Diet, I won't have to give up alcohol or desserts completely, because it allows them as occasional treats. And while I may feel miserable sometimes because I can't eat a pint of ice cream or drink a glass of chardonnay whenever I want, at other times I will probably feel fantastic because I will be losing weight. Skipping a sundae or a few glasses of wine may make me feel deprived in the moment, but fitting into a pair of pants that I haven't worn lately will make me feel great— and that feeling will last much longer than the enjoyment I would have felt from food or wine.

▶ **HURTFUL NEGATIVE THOUGHT**: Even if I can lose a few pounds, I'll still be overweight.

Helpful restructured thought: Sure, I'll still be overweight even if I lose a few pounds. But I'll be less overweight than I am now, and with even modest weight loss I will be lowering my risk of heart disease and other health problems. And if I lose a small amount of weight, it may motivate me to continue eating a healthy diet and being more active, which will allow me to lose even more weight.

▶ **HURTFUL NEGATIVE THOUGHT**: Losing weight is too hard. I'll never be able to succeed.

Helpful restructured thought: It's true that changing my diet and becoming more active may be difficult. But I've done lots of difficult things in my life, and I've succeeded at many of them. I am strong, and I can do hard things. And most of the time, the benefits will outweigh the sacrifices.

▶ **HURTFUL NEGATIVE THOUGHT**: I can't exercise because I don't like the way it feels to be sweaty and out of breath.

Helpful restructured thought: Exercise does not have to be intense to be useful, and I don't have to pant and sweat in order to move my body and increase my heart rate in a beneficial way. Dr. Juan says that walking at a moderate pace offers many benefits, and that as we become more active, our fitness level increases and we feel less out of breath. Maybe someday I'll want to do more strenuous exercise, but for now, I can do activities that won't cause me to get sweaty or out of breath.

Keep At It!

As you work on restructuring your automatic negative thoughts about weight loss, keep in mind that shifting your thought patterns isn't necessarily easy. Negative self-talk can be persistent, and when you consciously try to reframe it, your thoughts may argue with you a bit and try to convince you that they're logical and useful. I urge you to stick with it, though — keep identifying your automatic negative thoughts, keep challenging them for their accuracy and their helpfulness to you, keep consciously reframing them from hurtful to helpful. If you continue to practice this three-step process, you'll find that over time your negative self-talk will begin to fade, and positive thoughts will start to take its place. As this happens, your confidence in yourself will grow.

DR. JUAN'S WISDOM

DITCH THOSE REGRETS!

Even though regret is a normal human feeling that we all experience, I want you to try hard to let go of it, especially in relation to your weight. Rather than spending your energy feeling ashamed of the numbers you saw on the scale this morning or the fact that you weigh more than you'd like, try to focus on the present moment and your future, rather than the past.

No matter what you weigh, how high your blood pressure is, or what your cholesterol profile looks like, you still have time to make changes that can have a positive impact on your future health. Sure, you may feel discouraged if you're overweight or obese. But the fact that you're reading this book means you're taking the first important step toward a healthier future. That's cause for celebration, not regret.

As the saying goes, it's far better to look ahead and prepare than to look back and regret.

Other Ways to Shift Your Thinking

Because thoughts have such a profound impact on actions, I'd like to leave you with a few other ideas about how to shift your weight-loss mind-set so that your thought patterns are working with you rather than against you.

Speak kindly to yourself. Go back to your list of automatic negative thoughts, and imagine saying them to your friends. I don't think you would! We can be very cruel to ourselves, and we say things to ourselves that we wouldn't dare say to others. Listen to yourself, and when you notice that you're bullying yourself, tell that inner critic to shut up and stop. Replace those mean thoughts with kinder, more supportive thoughts.

Set your goal for control. Setting a goal and not meeting it can be discouraging, especially if you are working hard. That's why I encourage you to set goals that truly are within your control. Rather than deciding you're going to lose X number of pounds by a certain date—which is something you can't completely control—it's better to decide that you're going to follow your eating plan carefully and exercise thirty minutes a day, five days a week. Those goals are more within your control than the exact number of pounds you want to lose.

Ban negativity in yourself and others. As we discussed in this chapter, your own negative self-talk can interfere with your ability to lose weight. But negative talk from others can sabotage you as well. It's terribly hard to eat right or exercise when a friend or family member is talking trash to you about your choices. Maybe they're jealous that you're trying to improve your health, or maybe they just don't like it that you aren't eating the other half of the cake they bought. I saw this firsthand after I diagnosed my mother with diabetes and recommended that she lose weight. She took my advice very seriously and began losing weight right away. Unfortunately, as she started dropping pounds, a few friends commented that she looked "sick." Even though my mother was happy to be losing weight, she questioned herself and my advice because of the comments from her friends. Looking back, my mother realized that her friends were probably envious of her success. Not only did she lose twenty pounds in three months, but she lowered her HbA1c from 12.3 percent to 6.5 percent, which is an amazing improvement. Whatever the reason for other people's pessimism, if someone in your world is sending lots of negativity your way, speak up. Kindly explain why their words are hurtful to you, and ask them to stop. They may feel threatened by your decision to take care of yourself, and a few gentle words may turn them around. Who knows, maybe they'll want to do the Mojito Diet with you! If the negativity doesn't stop, speak to them again, and try to help them understand that you need their support, not their criticism. Then, if that doesn't work, seriously consider limiting your contact with them.

Get professional help if you need it. Sometimes negative self-talk is a sign of a more serious emotional problem or a psychological condition that you can't solve on your own, no matter how hard you try. That's okay. Help is available, and you don't have to suffer in silence. Speak to your family doctor, a therapist, a social worker, or a psychologist. And if you are in immediate distress or are having thoughts about harming yourself, call the National Suicide Prevention Lifeline at 800-273-8255 right away. Asking for help is a gift you can give yourself and your loved ones.

Commit to having a problem-solving attitude. Even though with the Mojito Diet I have created a program that gives you a step-by-step guide to eating a healthier diet and adding activity to your life, you may face challenges that aren't addressed in this book. Rather than allowing these challenges to derail your progress, try to adopt a problem-solving attitude that allows you to say, "No problem! I can figure this out!" rather than "Uh-oh. I give up." No matter how hard you try to keep your life under control, problems and difficulties arise—you come down with a cold that keeps you from exercising, perhaps, or you receive an invitation to a party with the most amazing dessert buffet you've ever seen. Don't give up—you can handle it! The more flexible you are about brainstorming potential solutions, the more likely you are to stick with your plan.

Use the thought of regret as a motivator. I started this chapter with a memory of all the regret I witnessed among heart attack victims who had undergone emergency cardiac catheterizations. If the challenge of losing a few pounds is weighing heavily on you, try to think of the people lying in intensive care units recuperating from heart attacks. They would give anything to trade places with you right now. They would love to be sitting in a comfortable chair reading a book, thinking about which recipe to cook for dinner, planning an after-dinner walk outdoors. It all comes down to perspective. You and I are the lucky ones, my friend.

DR. JUAN'S WISDOM

START WITH THE GREENS, AND OTHER BUFFET TIPS

Buffets present a loaded table of challenges to people who are trying to lose weight. But buffets are part of life, so the best way to deal with them is to think ahead and have a plan in place. Here are some ways to negotiate a buffet table without overeating:

▶ *Don't show up hungry.* Eat a high-protein, high-fiber snack (such as yogurt with berries, an apple with peanut butter, or whole grain crackers with cheese) before hitting the buffet. Without hunger pangs driving your choices, you'll be better able to stay away from high-calorie fare.

▶ *Start with the greens.* Fill your plate with raw spinach, baby kale, romaine, and other veggies. Dress them with a small amount of dressing. Fresh fruit is a good option, too, as long as it's not drenched in sugar syrup.

▶ *Take the edge off your hunger.* Sit down and eat your salad or fruit before going back for main dishes—that way you'll be less hungry when facing the heavier foods and will be better positioned to make smart choices.

▶ *Sit with your back to the buffet.* Out of sight, out of mind.

▶ *Choose "naked" proteins.* As much as possible, pick meat, poultry, and seafood that aren't swimming in butter or loaded with heavy sauces.

▶ *Skip the white pasta and white rice.* They're low-quality carbs that are most likely dripping with butter.

▶ *Take small portions.* Buffet food tends to be really high in calories and excess fat. Keeping portions small will help protect you from eating too much.

▶ *Ask about other options.* Some restaurants will allow you to skip the buffet and pick something healthier from the ordinary menu, such as baked fish and vegetables. It's worth asking.

▶ *Splurge judiciously.* Let's face it, the food on most buffets isn't that great. It's chosen because it feeds a crowd and holds up well under heat lamps. If there really is something amazing on the buffet, go ahead and treat yourself to it. But really, the chances of finding something amazing on a buffet are pretty slim.

MOJITO DIET SUCCESS STORY: **DANA**

Losing Weight During Menopause

Dana put on some extra weight as she went through menopause. That's not unusual—the hormonal shifts that occur during menopause can lead to stubborn weight gain of ten pounds or more, including excess fat around the belly. Menopausal weight gain can be so frustrating for women, because it seems sometimes that no matter what they do, they can't rid themselves of those extra pounds. Many just give up, which leads to even more weight gain.

A change in medication also contributed to excess weight for Dana, a fifty-five-year-old dentist.

Dana tried to lose weight through various strategies, including low-carb diets, commercial weight-loss plans, meal replacement programs, and food delivery systems, but none of them worked. She actually gained weight, rather than losing it, while following a paleo-style plan.

Although she felt frustrated, Dana refused to give up. "I wanted to lose weight for three reasons," Dana says. "I wanted to return to better health, I wanted to feel better, because I was feeling the burden of the added weight, and I wanted to improve my appearance."

As it turns out, the Mojito Diet was the plan that finally worked for Dana. In fifteen weeks she lost nineteen pounds and went down two pants sizes.

Success feels sweet for Dana. "I had been exercising before, but now I'm better able to handle aerobic exercise and I'm in much better shape," Dana says. "I liked the ease of the Mojito Diet. The structure was important, and I like that it combines the best practices of several different types of diets."

Dana also appreciated that the Mojito Diet left space for alcohol. "I don't generally drink but allowing the mojito reward is important for that occasional event where I do have a drink."

3

~~~~~~~

Have a Mojito: How to Use Rewards to Help with Weight Loss

Why do I include mojitos in my weight-loss plan? Why do I consider them to be such an important part of my diet that I have included them in its name? Because I don't believe in deprivation! Many diets tell you that you can never drink alcohol or never eat cake or never have bread or a long list of other foods and drinks. But I believe that deprivation doesn't work, and that the path to long-term weight-loss success includes occasional indulgences.

My patients don't believe in deprivation either. "Don't tell me I can't have a cocktail when I go to a restaurant or a party!" they often say when I talk with them about losing weight. "We live in Miami, for goodness' sake! I can't give up my favorite cocktail!"

As a weight-loss strategy, deprivation can work temporarily, but it rarely holds up over time. Depriving yourself of the foods and drinks you enjoy is unpleasant—I believe it's one of the reasons that people are so unwilling to try to lose weight in the first place, and why many give up on their weight-loss plans after a week or two. I see it in my practice all the time. When I talk with overweight or obese patients about trying to drop a few pounds, they tell me they can't bear the thought of having to give up alcohol or red meat or bread or fruit or other favorites. They don't want to eliminate specific foods or entire food groups from their lives. They are so thrilled when I tell them that they can succeed without taking such an all-or-nothing approach, using a strategy based on moderation rather than deprivation.

Trying to eliminate specific foods from your diet long-term can backfire. I don't know about you, but nothing makes me think about something more than being told I shouldn't think about it at all! Tell me I can never have bread again, and I'll probably start dreaming about it at night. Sure, there are some foods that you are better off cutting back on. But to say that you can never have them again will just make you crave them more. There's nothing you *can't* eat on the Mojito Diet.

In the Mojito Diet, I do sometimes ask you to temporarily eliminate certain foods from your diet. For example, during my Week 1 Grain Drop, I recommend cutting out all grains. I do this to help give you a big boost when you begin your weight-loss plan. However, during the Week 2 Clean 16 Fast, you can start eating bread, cereal, rice, tortillas, and other grains again.

Deprivation diets that never allow certain foods feel like punishment. They can make you feel miserable and angry—and who wants to feel miserable and angry? I don't, and I don't think you do either. And I know my patients don't—they have made that very clear to me! Diets that forbid occasional treats such as alcohol or dessert don't take into account the fact that enjoying these special pleasures can be an important part of the social events that are so meaningful to us. Respecting and encouraging people's social interactions and cultural traditions is important to me, because I recognize how important social support is to our health. Many studies have linked strong social support to better health, including heart health. Having people we love around us isn't just a nicety—it truly does our hearts good.

I'm not saying that if you don't drink alcohol you can't enjoy going to parties or socializing with your family and friends. Many people live very happy lives without drinking a drop of alcohol. I don't drink at all when I'm on call, because as a physician I don't want to be in any way impaired when my patients need me. On those occasions when I'm not drinking alcohol, I have just as much fun at parties and social events.

Even when I'm not on duty, I drink only in moderation—I love mojitos and like to enjoy myself, but have no intention of ever letting alcohol ruin my health. Despite my best efforts, my blood sugar can rise higher than I'd like, and alcohol raises it even more, so I am happy with moderation.

If alcohol is an enjoyable part of your life, and if your doctor has not recommended that you give up alcohol for health reasons, then you can continue to enjoy it in moderation. The Mojito Diet makes strategic use of mojitos (or other alcoholic beverages or desserts) as occasional rewards. If you choose not to drink, you can have occasional desserts instead. Although I do ask you to be judicious and moderate with alcohol and desserts, I won't ask you to deprive yourself.

Alcohol and Heart Health

We hear a lot of talk about moderate alcohol use being heart-healthy. But is that true? Is alcohol really good for your heart? The answer to that question is yes. And no. Either one can be true, depending on your own health history and a few other factors.

First, let's look at the possible benefits of drinking alcohol. Whenever a study is published linking alcohol to health, big headlines appear in the news. Most of the positive research about alcohol and heart health pertains to red wine, although some studies have found health advantages with other kinds of alcohol as well. Red wine contains antioxidants, which are substances that help protect your cells, and resveratrol, a natural chemical that has been linked to heart health. Some studies have found that drinking red wine helps increase HDL ("good") cholesterol and may help keep platelets in your blood from sticking together and contributing to heart attack and stroke. I've seen enough studies linking red wine and heart health to believe there is a connection.

However, we don't know exactly *how* they are linked. Many of the red wine–drinking populations that have been studied, such as people living in the Mediterranean, also do other things that benefit their hearts, such as exercising; eating a diet rich in heart-healthy foods such as fruits, vegetables, healthy fats, and nuts; and spending lots of time with their support network of friends and family. It's notoriously hard for researchers to tease out the specific causes of health benefits in populations with multiple wellness habits.

My father-in-law is from Spain, and he believes that red wine is the cure for everything! Anytime he has gone on medication, such as cholesterol medicine, his first question to me has always been, "Can I drink red wine while on this drug?" I'm actually not sure why he even asks me this, because I'm pretty sure he wouldn't stop drinking his beloved red wine even if I told him to!

Beyond red wine, studies suggest that drinking other kinds of alcohol may be beneficial as well. For example, a four-year study of more than two million adults in England, which was published in 2017 in the prestigious journal *BMJ*, found that moderate drinkers were less likely to experience certain heart and blood vessel diseases than those who never drank alcohol.

Reading that might make you think you should drink more—or, if you don't drink, that you should start. But I warn you not to jump to that conclusion. Even moderate drinking does have some risks—for example, researchers believe that moderate drinking can increase the likelihood of some types of cancer. And you can get the heart-health benefits of alcohol from other sources. The antioxidants and resveratrol in red wine, for instance, can also be found in foods such as fruits (especially berries) and vegetables. And taking a daily aspirin may lower the risk of heart attack and stroke in certain people.

One thing we absolutely know for sure is that drinking more than a moderate amount of alcohol is not good for your health. (The American Heart Association defines "moderate drinking" as one to two drinks per day for men, and one drink per day for women. However, I recommend less than that—I'll come back to that in a minute.) Drinking more than a moderate amount of alcohol raises the risk of all kinds of problems, including alcoholism, accidents, and suicide, as well as high blood pressure, stroke, heart failure, obesity, breast cancer, and diabetes. Excess alcohol can increase triglycerides, and can boost the likelihood of irregular heartbeat, heart muscle disease, and sudden cardiac death. There's no doubt about it: drinking excessively is all kinds of bad.

Here's where I stand on this question. Because you can get the heart-health benefits of alcohol from other sources, such as healthy foods and exercise, I don't recommend that you drink simply to help your heart. If you don't drink, there's no need to start for the sake of your heart. But if you do enjoy drinking in moderation and your doctor has no objection to it, it's fine to have an occasional mixed drink, glass of wine, or beer.

> *What are you drinking? Share your mojito reward on social media! Post a photo of your mojito with the hashtag #mojitodiet! And be sure to tag me @drjuanjr on Instagram or Twitter!*

What Does *Moderation* Mean?

Before we go any further, let's talk a little about the word *moderation*. As I said before, the American Heart Association considers "moderate drinking" to be one drink per day for women, and one to two drinks per day for men. However, to my mind, that's too much alcohol. I recommend limiting alcohol to two drinks *per week*—not per day—if you're trying to lose weight, and three drinks per week if you're maintaining weight loss. (If you're substituting desserts for mojitos, the same guidelines apply. A serving of dessert is one small slice of cake, one or two cookies, one small serving of flan, or other sweets or treats with a count of under 200 calories.)

Here's the thinking behind my alcohol recommendations. Having one or two drinks a day is a lot when you're trying to lose weight or maintain weight loss. Depending on what you choose, a drink delivers somewhere in the neighborhood of 125 to several hundred calories. We don't really focus on calories in the Mojito Diet, but it's helpful to think about them when discussing alcohol. If you're trying to lose weight or avoid weight gain, the math just doesn't work out in your favor if you're consuming one or two drinks each day. It's easier to meet your weight goals with fewer drinks, and it's better to use your calories eating healthier foods.

I also notice that people who have a drink or two every day also tend to eat more—not necessarily because they're hungrier, but because alcohol affects their ability to make smart choices about what and how much they eat. Even though alcohol contains calories, your body doesn't recognize and become satiated by them as it does with food calories—in fact, I think that alcohol actually makes you hungrier. If you've ever eaten half a jar of cocktail nuts or a giant plate of nachos after having a few drinks, you know what I mean.

Another thing happens when people have one drink a day. It's very easy for that one drink to become two drinks or three drinks. You and your spouse may plan on having just one glass of wine each, but it's easy to have a little more, and before you know it, the whole bottle is gone. And maybe the cork on a second bottle is popped.

I think of alcohol as an occasional indulgence, something to look forward to a couple of times per week. Having it every day takes away its specialness, and turns it from a reward to a habit. Limiting alcohol to two or three times per week allows you to enjoy it without letting it sabotage your weight-loss efforts or interfere with your health.

DR. JUAN'S WISDOM

KNOW HOW MUCH YOU'RE DRINKING

Just as it's important to measure your food to make sure you're getting the right-size portions, it's also smart to pay attention to portion sizes with alcohol. One serving of alcohol is:

- ▶ 12 ounces of beer (with a 5 percent alcohol content)

- ▶ 8 ounces of malt liquor (with a 7 percent alcohol content)

- ▶ 5 ounces of wine (with a 12 percent alcohol content)

- ▶ 1 shot (1.5 ounces) distilled spirits such as rum, gin, whiskey, or vodka

Alcohol Isn't for Everyone

For reasons of health and safety, some people should not drink alcohol. Your doctor can help you decide whether you should abstain, but in general, as I tell my patients, do not drink if you:

■ *Have been told by your doctor to avoid alcohol for other reasons.* For example, your doctor may prefer that you abstain if you have diabetes and high blood pressure, or if you take daily aspirin for heart health and have gastrointestinal problems.

■ *Take prescription or over-the-counter medications that interact with alcohol in an unhealthy way.* Alcohol may interact harmfully with more than a hundred medications, according to the National Institute on Alcohol Abuse and Alcoholism. If you have any questions at all about whether you can drink alcohol while taking a medication, talk with your doctor.

■ *Have certain health conditions that can be worsened by alcohol.* These include liver disease (cirrhosis, hepatitis B or C), mental health disorders (including anxiety, depression, post-traumatic stress disorder, schizophrenia), certain immune system diseases, heart failure, and high blood pressure, to name just a few.

■ *Have a drinking problem.* It's important for you to avoid alcohol of any kind if you are unable to control your drinking or are recovering from alcoholism, or if drinking causes you to become violent or to have trouble with your family, friends, job, or school.

■ *Are a woman who is pregnant or is planning to become pregnant.* Drinking alcohol during pregnancy can cause serious health problems, including premature birth, brain damage, birth defects, low birth weight, miscarriage, stillbirth, and fetal alcohol syndrome. No amount of alcohol is considered safe at any time during pregnancy. Because most women don't know they are pregnant until four to six weeks into their pregnancy, and because half of all pregnancies in the United States are unplanned, it's best to avoid alcohol if you're trying to get pregnant or if you are not using effective birth control.

▪ *Intend to get behind the wheel.* Alcohol is one of the top causes of car crashes in the United States. Don't drink if you're going to drive, use machinery, or engage in any type of activity that requires concentration and alertness.

▪ *Have survived or are at high risk for certain cancers.* Several kinds of cancers have been linked to alcohol intake, so you may want to abstain or limit alcohol if you are a survivor of or at high risk for developing cancer of the breast, mouth, pharynx, larynx, esophagus, liver, colon, or rectum.

Mindful Mojitos

Whether you decide to reward yourself with mojitos or desserts while following the Mojito Diet, I hope that you will engage in a practice known as mindfulness while you enjoy them. Mindfulness can increase exponentially the pleasure of a celebratory mojito, a favorite dessert, or any delicious food or drink.

Being mindful means paying attention to the here and now, and making an effort to be fully aware of what is unfolding in the present, rather than being distracted by thoughts of the past or future. Engaging in mindful eating and mindful drinking allows you to apply this kind of present-tense living to food and drink.

When mojito time rolls around, don't just chug it down like a bottle of water at the end of a three-mile run along the Miami Beach Boardwalk. Slow down. Enjoy it. Savor it. Use all of your senses to be mindful of it.

So often our minds are on autopilot, rushing from one thought to another in a reactionary way. Rather than thinking about what you're doing at this moment, you look back ("Did yesterday's meeting go well?" "Why did my husband snap at me this morning?" "Did my boss notice I was late for work this morning?") or you look ahead ("I have to remember to buy milk on the way home from the office today." "Will I be able to finish my work on time?" "I wonder if the car needs new tires?").

When you practice mindfulness, you choose to be aware of what is occurring in this moment, rather than allowing your mind to race with thoughts and concerns about the past and future. You let go of worries and cares about what has already happened or what will happen, and focus instead on what is happening right now. Being mindful during any activity—work, sex, exercise, eating—can help sharpen your focus and enhance your enjoyment of what you're doing. And by concentrating on the present moment, you can help block out some of the worries that may cause stress and anxiety.

When you eat mindfully, you choose to direct your attention to what you are eating or drinking so that you can fully appreciate and take pleasure from it. Instead of rushing, you slow down and use all of your senses to observe, identify, and savor the aroma, taste, texture, and temperature of your food.

Imagine drinking a mojito with mindfulness. You feel the frosty coldness of the glass in your hand, see the shape of the glass and the bright green of the fresh mint in the drink, smell the aromas of lime and mint and rum, hear the clink of ice and fizzy pops of seltzer bubbles, and then, as you taste your first sip, feel the icy sensation on your lips and taste the fresh flavors of the cold drink on your tongue. Then you sit back and relax.

Now imagine expanding that mindfulness beyond the mojito you're drinking. Extend your awareness to what's going on around you—the people you're with, the enjoyment you feel while relaxing after a long day, the fulfillment you experience as you look around at your family and think about how proud of them you are, even the pleasure you feel as you observe and appreciate what you see before you, such as the living room you recently painted or the view outside your window.

In Miami we love to sit outside and enjoy our view of the shimmering ocean, white sand beaches, and swaying palm trees—or the people walking by. But even if your view isn't postcard-worthy, it can still be awe-inspiring if you slow down and take time to savor it with mindfulness and appreciation. A good friend of mine who lives in New England loves to bundle up, sit on the deck in her backyard, and have a glass of champagne with her husband during the first snowfall of winter each year. She says that taking time to enjoy and celebrate the beauty of that first snowfall helps take away some of the sting of having to shovel!

A Way to Slow Down

Practicing mindful eating or drinking slows you down, pulls your attention away from the millions of other thoughts running around in your head, and gives you the space to appreciate what you're consuming. How often have you zoomed through a meal or a beverage and barely remembered having it? When you eat or drink mindlessly, you miss an opportunity for enjoyment and pleasure. You also are likely to eat or drink more than you intended, because your food or beverage scarcely registers in your mind as it zips through your mouth and down into your stomach. Because your attention is diverted, you risk eating or drinking too much.

Eating more slowly gives your body time to recognize that you are taking in calories, and to alert you when your hunger begins to subside. When you bolt down your food or drink, you are likely to eat more than you need because the biochemical communication between your stomach and your brain doesn't have time to work properly.

Mindful eating isn't just for special, celebratory foods. In fact, employing mindful eating can be an excellent way to rediscover the deliciousness of everyday foods and the healthy foods you may now be choosing to eat without added sugar or salt. For example, try eating an apple mindfully and you'll probably find it much more enjoyable than you do when you munch apples thoughtlessly. Observe the apple's color and shine, feel its smooth firmness in your hand, hear the snap of the knife as you slice through the apple's skin and flesh, enjoy its earthy aroma, feel the crunch of the fruit on your teeth as you take a bite, taste the tart-sweet flavor of the apple's juice on your tongue and the crispness of the flesh as you chew. When you eat a food with mindfulness—even an ordinary food that you have eaten a million times—you can appreciate and enjoy it fully. By increasing your awareness of what you are consuming, you are more likely to feel satisfied by a reasonable serving size and less likely to eat more than you want.

Eating and drinking mindfully also offers an opportunity to feel gratitude for your food. As you eat your apple, think of the creator who made it and all the people who worked to bring it to you—the farmer who grew it, the laborer who picked it, the trucker who drove it to your town, the grocery store worker who unpacked and displayed it, and the person who shopped for it (especially if it wasn't you!). Gratitude is a powerful emotion, and inviting it into your mind can enhance your appreciation of your food and your life. It can also help put weight loss into perspective. Yes, it's important to try to lose weight to improve your health—but in the grand scheme of things, appreciating the gifts we've been given and making the most of our time with family and friends are what truly bring us happiness.

Setting Goals and Choosing Rewards

The Mojito Diet includes occasional alcoholic beverages or desserts so that you can continue to enjoy those pleasures while still losing weight. However, there are many other nonfood and nonalcoholic treats and rewards you can give yourself while following a weight-loss plan. In fact, setting goals and planning on rewarding yourself when you reach them can be very inspiring and can help lead you to success.

Rewards and incentives give you something to work toward, and are a great way to celebrate when you achieve a goal or reach a milestone. As you begin the Mojito Diet, I suggest that you think about your goals for weight loss and health, and use them to fuel your motivation. Use these guidelines to help you plan goals and rewards that will bring you success.

Write a weight-loss mission statement

Take some time to sit down and really think about why you want to lose weight. Is it just about how you look, or are you thinking about specific health goals, such as lowering your blood pressure or controlling your blood sugar? Your motivation matters, because by fully understanding what lies behind your desire to lose weight, you can create a day-to-day strategy that will help you succeed.

To explore your motivations, spend time journaling or sitting quietly and visualizing what success would look like for you. Ask yourself: What do I want to achieve? What is most important to me? Why does it matter? Once you have a clear picture of what you want, write it down in the form of a mission statement that spells out your overarching goal and the reason you want to achieve it. For example: "My mission is to be healthier, feel more energetic, and lose weight. I will follow the Mojito Diet and be more active every day. By taking these steps, I hope to improve my heart health and lose 5 percent of my body weight." Consider posting your mission statement in a place where you'll see it often, such as the mirror you look into every morning as you put on your makeup or shave.

Break your big goal into smaller goals

After determining your big-picture goal, think about what you must do on a daily basis to make it happen. What will you do every day and every week to align you with your mission? What actions belong on your daily to-do list? Use specifics as you set goals. Rather than "I will exercise more," say "I will exercise for twenty to thirty minutes at least four days a week." Put your goals in writing, and read them every day.

Set realistic weight goals

This is the place where most diet books would tell you how much weight you *should* lose. They would present you with a body mass index (BMI) chart, and you would use your height and your current weight to determine how overweight you are and how much weight you should try to lose. I'm not going to give you one of those charts, though. Why? Because if you're overweight or obese, you already know it. And you already know that losing some weight would improve your health.

I believe that for most people, getting too hung up on numbers at this point can be discouraging, rather than motivating. And so, instead of obsessing over numbers, let's do this. If you really want to figure out your perfect goal weight, google the words "Calculate Your Body Mass Index NIH" and use the handy BMI calculator from the National Institutes of Health. Otherwise, let's just have you start off by aiming to lose 5 to 7 percent of your body weight, since studies have shown that a weight loss of that proportion can bring about a reduction in the risk of type 2 diabetes and heart disease. Achieving that would give you some great potential health benefits without making you feel discouraged or overwhelmed.

Here's how to figure out your Mojito Diet first-step goal weight: Simply take your current weight and multiply it by 0.05 (for a 5 percent weight loss), and again by 0.07 (for a 7 percent weight loss). Here's an example for someone who weighs 200 pounds:

- 5 percent weight loss: 200 x 0.05 = 10 pounds

- 7 percent weight loss: 200 x 0.07 = 14 pounds

Then, once you lose 5 to 7 percent of your current weight, you can reset your goal and lose an additional 5 to 7 percent of your new weight, if you'd like. In my experience, you're more likely to reach big, long-term goals by breaking them up into smaller, less intimidating mini-goals.

DR. JUAN'S WISDOM

PREP FOR SUCCESS

Once you've got your weight-loss and exercise goals figured out, think about what you need to do to smooth your pathway to success. A new pair of supportive sneakers for your daily walks? A new kitchen scale to measure serving sizes accurately? Would it be easier for you to attend that yoga class if your husband drives the kids to school instead of you doing it? Should you throw away that stash of Halloween candy hidden in the kitchen cabinet so you're not tempted to snack on it? Taking steps like those can make it easier for you to go after your goals.

Choose attainable goals

Trying to achieve unrealistic goals simply sets you up for disappointment and failure. You're more likely to stick with your plan when you choose goals you can truly attain. For example, if you've been overweight for decades, deciding that you're going to whittle yourself down to what you weighed on your wedding day may be too much of a challenge; trying to get there may frustrate you so much that you'll give up during your first week. Instead, start with a more modest, achievable goal—perhaps half of the amount you've gained since your walk down the aisle.

Do what's within your control

By focusing your daily and weekly goals on performance rather than outcome, you have more chance of long-term success. For example, rather than tell yourself you're going to lose three pounds this week, decide instead that this week you will follow the Mojito Diet as closely as possible and will be active twenty minutes per day. You can control what you eat and how active you are (your performance), but you can't necessarily control the specific outcome (the numbers on the scale) on a daily or weekly basis.

Think about your dreams too

As long as you choose attainable, realistic goals, you can expect to achieve them, especially if you define an action plan that aligns your daily choices with your goals. However, there is a difference between goals and dreams. Dreams are not quite as attainable—in fact, they may seem nearly impossible. But that doesn't mean you shouldn't dream! Your dreams can inspire you, even if you don't have a clue how you might make them happen.

For example, you may dream of running a marathon or hiking the Appalachian Trail or climbing Mount Everest. When you write down your mission statement, make a note of your dreams too. But start with your goals. Work on achieving them and making yourself stronger and healthier. Then someday you may be in a position to turn your dreams into goals.

My dream is to be a singer, so I sing in the shower every day—my kids have even recorded me. One time I sang with mariachis on Univision's morning show, but quite frankly, it was disastrous. I will never be a professional singer, but you better believe that I will continue singing in the shower no matter how hard my kids laugh at me. Get the point? Keep pushing, keep grinding—yes, it's true that I will never sing professionally, but it makes my showers more enjoyable! Maybe you won't ever fit into your wedding dress again, but the day-to-day effort to lose weight and get healthier will make you feel like a newlywed again.

Choose rewards that align with your goals

Now the fun part: What will you do to celebrate your success when you meet specific goals? Rewards can be an excellent motivator. I recommend that you designate specific rewards for specific actions. For example, tell yourself that if you are active for twenty minutes on each of five days this week, you will treat yourself to a new pair of sunglasses. Or decide that after following the Mojito Diet as closely as possible for three weeks, you'll have a massage. Here are some ideas for rewards that help keep you motivated: a new puppy (don't tell my daughter I said that, though), a book by your favorite author (and a quiet afternoon for reading), a bubble bath, a day at a spa, a day pass at a fancy gym, a manicure or pedicure—or how about a weekend in Miami Beach!

Plan to reevaluate your mission statement and your goals

I encourage you to revisit your mission statement and your daily and weekly goals, and revise them as needed, especially if they're too easy or too difficult. Goals can also be rewritten when you reach certain milestones. For example, if you plan to walk a mile a day, you may choose to increase your goal to two miles a day when you start walking faster and getting fitter.

Be kind to yourself

My final piece of advice is not to be too hard on yourself. Setting goals is important, and of course you want to commit to them and try to achieve them. But sometimes things won't go exactly as you planned, and that's okay. We're all human, and we all make mistakes. There will be days when you won't live up to your own expectations. When that happens, thank yourself for trying. Acknowledge that what you're trying to do isn't easy, but it's so worthwhile. Forgive yourself for missing the mark. And then take a deep breath and resolve to do better tomorrow.

DR. JUAN'S WISDOM

BUILD YOURSELF A TEAM

Just as you can be dragged down by negativity and pessimism in others, you can be lifted up by positivity and optimism. I urge you to gather a team of positive, supportive people who are enthusiastic about your weight-loss goals, who are willing to cheer you on when you're doing great, and who will help pull you up when you're feeling down. Tell your team about your weight-loss plan, and ask them to be there for you when you need them. (And offer to return the favor if they want to do the Mojito Diet with you.)

Studies have found that social support can have a hugely positive impact on weight loss. It doesn't matter whether you communicate with your cheerleaders in person, by phone, or online. Positive support can make your weight-loss journey so much more enjoyable and successful, so seek it out wherever you can find it.

MOJITO DIET SUCCESS STORY: ANA

Exercising Five Times a Week But Not Losing Pounds

Ana's main incentive for trying the Mojito Diet was to see better results from all of the effort she was putting into her workouts. Although Ana, twenty-four, who works as a digital media manager, was going to the gym three to five times a week, she wasn't losing weight. "I realized that I had to eat a balanced diet too," Ana says.

Ana's weight started to go down as soon as she began following the Mojito Diet, and in one month she dropped fifteen pounds and trimmed three inches off her waistline. Slimming down energized Ana because it allowed her to really see the positive impact that her fitness regimen was having on her body.

And she saw an unexpected benefit too: After starting the Mojito Diet, Ana began to sleep better.

Although Ana has been trying to eat healthier during the past couple of years, this was the first time she's followed a formal diet plan. "I had a positive and eye-opening experience with the Mojito Diet," Ana says. "The Mojito Diet gave me the structure I needed. It forced me to think about the portions of food—and drinks—I was putting into my body. It taught me that moderation is the key to results and maintaining a healthy lifestyle."

Ana appreciates that the Mojito Diet isn't too strict and makes room for alcohol. "Most diets restrict your foods too much and completely rule out alcohol by any means," Ana says. "I wanted a diet that I could stick with for the long term and truly enjoy its process. I did not want a diet that I would dread to begin and count the hours until it was over."

When she first started following the Mojito Diet, Ana kept track of her daily portions on her cell phone so she could reference them at any moment. But now she knows them by heart and has a good visual understanding of how much food she should be eating each day. Ana says, "This diet has become an essential tool in my life, and I plan on using it for years to come."

4

Feel the Rhythm with the Mojito Diet Exercise Plan

Sometimes my patients ask me if they have to exercise. Can't they lose weight without it? The answer is yes—while it is easier to lose weight if you combine a healthy diet with daily activity, it's also true that you can lower your weight without doing any exercise at all. But, my friend, if this is your plan, I beg you to reconsider. Exercise is so good for you and has so many health benefits that if we could put all those health benefits into a pill, it would be the most prescribed medication in the entire world. Exercise helps us in so many ways that if it were a drug, it would be hailed as a miracle, and people would be lined up outside their doctors' offices to get a prescription.

Activity doesn't just help with weight loss. It also lowers the risk of dozens—maybe even hundreds—of health conditions and diseases, including nearly all of the chronic conditions that hold a place on the list of leading causes of death in the United States. Exercise can extend life as well as improving it. Research published in 2012 found that regular exercise added between two and seven years of life for study participants. Crunching those numbers leads to a pretty amazing conclusion: For the people in the study, which followed more than 650,000 adults of all ages for ten years, every minute of exercise was linked to as much as seven extra minutes of life.

The most effective way to lose weight and keep it off for good is to combine a healthy diet with activities that burn calories and strengthen your heart and lungs. You can do any kind of activities you want—walking, swimming, jogging, playing tennis, or anything else—but if you want to have a huge amount of fun, I heartily recommend that you take up salsa dancing.

Wait a minute. You may be thinking that you don't know how to dance, or that you don't like dancing—after all, you tried it in high school and felt like a fool. Or you took a ballroom dancing class before your wedding and never could get the hang of it because you have two left feet. Or you think you're too old, too overweight, too uncoordinated, or too shy to learn to dance. Or you have nobody to dance with.

If any of those thoughts come to mind in relation to dancing, let me tell you: You're wrong, wrong, wrong, wrong, wrong. And wrong again! If you think you don't like dancing, or that you can't do it, you've probably never tried salsa dancing. It is one of the most enjoyable activities you can imagine—and anyone can do it! If you can walk, you can dance the salsa. And if you like the idea of having so much fun while you're doing a fitness activity that you forget that what you're doing is exercise, you have to give salsa dancing a try.

In Miami, salsa dancing breaks out at parties, weddings, family celebrations, and just about any other gathering at which there are people and music. I love seeing friends and family members of all ages and all sizes salsa dancing together, laughing and enjoying each other and moving their bodies. Walk down Ocean Drive or Collins Avenue in Miami Beach nearly any evening of the week, and you'll hear the percussive beat of salsa music (a rhythm pattern known as the clave) flowing from the many dance clubs that draw so many people to our city. It's nearly impossible to see people salsa dancing or to hear salsa music and not want to join in!

BEFORE YOU START MOVING

Keep these tips in mind as you make your exercise plan.

▶ *Check in with your doctor.* Moderate-intensity exercise is safe for most people, even those with chronic health conditions. But it's important to get your doctor's okay before starting to exercise, especially if you have health problems or have been inactive in the past.

▶ *Exercise safely.* Be sure to follow all safety rules related to your activity. For example, wear a helmet for cycling, and dress in light colors when walking at night. And follow any health guidelines your doctor may recommend. For instance, a doctor may advise someone with high blood pressure to avoid lifting heavy weights and stick to lighter weights. If you have diabetes, your doctor may recommend that you eat something before exercising to avoid hypoglycemia. No problem—just find out what you have to do, and do it.

▶ *Equip yourself.* No need to spend a lot of money on trendy fitness wear, but it is important to wear clothing and shoes that are supportive and comfortable for whatever activity you choose. (For best results and optimal safety, choose shoes designed for your activity, such as walking shoes or running shoes.) And keep in mind that exercise warms you up, so dressing in layers will allow you to cool down as your heart rate goes up.

▶ *Take it easy.* If you are sedentary and rarely exercise, it's not a great idea to jump in and try to do a vigorous one-hour exercise class. If you do, you risk walking away from it (or, more likely, limping away) feeling sore and discouraged. Go at a pace that is safe for you, and increase intensity as you become more fit.

▶ *Stay hydrated.* Drink water before, during, and after exercise.

▶ *Keep trying new activities until you find one you love.* In addition to salsa dancing and brisk walking, you can try jogging, water aerobics, tennis, biking, hiking, swimming, playing basketball, or any other activity or sport. Or mix them up and do something different every week.

Exercising Joy

What I love most about salsa dancing as a physical activity is that it is so pleasurable. My patients sometimes complain that exercise feels more like drudgery than fun—if you've ever watched minute after minute after minute drag by on a treadmill or stationary bike, you know what I mean. But salsa dancing is so enjoyable that it's easy to lose track of time as you immerse yourself in music and movement. At dance clubs in Miami, people salsa dance for hours at a time, and when the last song of the night plays they're shocked that the evening flew by so quickly!

Enjoying the physical activities that you choose to do is important because it's just too hard to stay committed to exercise that you don't like. Life is too short to force yourself to jog when you hate it or to try to power through a half hour of lap swimming every day if you dislike going in the water. I always say that if you ask Latinos to run a marathon at 6 a.m., very few of us would be there; but invite us to an afternoon salsa festival, and we all show up and stay for hours dancing our asses off.

I've seen it time and time again with my patients: When they attempt to do a fitness activity they don't enjoy, they drop it within weeks or even days of starting. It's too hard to do something they dislike. That's why I encourage you to try salsa dancing. Dancers give their hearts a workout—in fact, salsa dancing can burn as many calories as jogging or swimming laps—but I think it's a lot more fun.

All dancing provides a great workout, but salsa dancing is especially good for fitness. In salsa, you typically keep your upper body level while you move your hips, legs, and feet. This provides you with multiple physical benefits: Vigorous movement gives you a cardio workout by causing your heart to beat faster to speed up blood flow throughout your body, and maintaining a level upper body helps strengthen the muscles in your core (abdomen, back, and pelvis). And as you move your lower body, you work the muscles in your hips and legs. Dancing also helps improve flexibility and balance, which is important at any age, but especially as we get older. Salsa dancing really is a full-body workout.

One of the great things about salsa dancing is you can do it anytime, anywhere. In Miami you sometimes see people doing dance moves on the street as they walk, or while they wait for a bus. It's fun to go to a club and dance, but you can dance at home too. Salsa dancing is an excellent home workout because it's so easy to do—load some salsa tunes on your smartphone, put on your earbuds, and dance for ten minutes. It's that easy. And if you want to see some big-time salsa moves, show up on a Friday afternoon at Estefan Kitchen, the restaurant owned by my good friends Gloria and Emilio Estefan in the Miami design district. You will see some jaw-dropping salsa moves from couples of all ages. And while you are at it, please have one of Estefan Kitchen's fabulous mojitos. They are the best!

DR. JUAN'S WISDOM

START WHEREVER YOU ARE

Sometimes when I advise my patients to start exercising, they become embarrassed. "I can't join a gym, Dr. Juan! I'm too out of shape!" Don't give in to that kind of thinking! And don't be ashamed to start where you are, even if you are totally out of shape or have never ever exercised before. If you're starting an exercise plan for the first time ever, you should be enormously proud, not embarrassed. Lift your head high, take pride in yourself, and go for it! I know it takes courage, but I also know that you are stronger than you realize. And I know that whenever I see someone in my gym who is very overweight or obviously out of shape, I don't judge them—I feel thrilled that they are stepping out of their comfort zone and into a healthier future!

It's perfectly fine to start slowly and increase your time and intensity gradually. If all you can do right now is walk slowly for five minutes, then walk slowly for five minutes. Do it every day, and before you know it, you'll be able to walk for ten minutes. And then fifteen minutes. The same is true with salsa dancing or Zumba classes or any other activity. Don't feel bad about yourself if you can't keep up with everyone else. Be true to yourself—the best place to start is exactly where you are right now. Go at your own pace, have faith that you'll get fitter over time, and celebrate the fact that you're moving.

Learning to Salsa Dance

I can't teach you salsa dancing moves in a book, but I can give you ideas about how to learn to salsa dance on your own. And I can guarantee that even if you have no dancing experience, you can learn salsa.

A great way to start picking up salsa dancing steps is with YouTube videos or DVDs. You can get started right away—just put on a video and follow along. Don't worry if it takes a while to catch on. What matters to your heart and your muscles is that you're moving your body, not that you're performing perfect choreography. Forget about whether your steps are just right—instead, practice mindfulness and use all of your senses to appreciate what you're doing. Enjoy the sound of the music, the energy you feel in your muscles as they wake up and start moving, and the smile on your face as you put aside the stresses of the day to focus on doing something just for you, something that gets you up and out of your chair. Sing along with the music if you'd like! Snap your fingers and move your hips! Pretend that you're Gloria Estefan or Marc Anthony! Celebrate that you're alive and that you're giving your body the gift of movement.

Another way to learn salsa dancing is by taking dance classes. In cities around the country, dance clubs offer lessons and Latin dance parties for people of all levels of experience. Some places schedule group dance lessons early in the evening or on weeknights, before the more serious dance crowd arrives. Lessons are usually free or inexpensive. Do a Google search for "salsa dance lessons" and the name of your city or town, and you'll probably be surprised by how many options there are.

Latin dance and salsa classes can also be found at local dance studios, community education centers, fitness centers, and health clubs, many of which have discovered that salsa dancing offers a fantastic mix of fun and fitness for people of all ages. You may even find Latin dancing fitness classes at your local hospital's patient education department.

Like other types of Latin dancing, salsa is usually done with a partner, but if you're solo, don't worry about it. Salsa dancing is social by nature, so most clubs and classes will match you with a partner if you show up without one. And at home, you can dance by yourself. You and your new friends can create your own Mojito Diet salsa group, and drink your reward mojitos to the beat of salsa music!

If you find you enjoy salsa dancing, you may also warm up to other dance styles, such as flamenco, ballroom, tap, swing, hip-hop, square dancing, contra dancing, line dancing, tango, merengue, soca, samba, or mambo. Once you start dancing, it's hard to stop!

Zumba and Other Dance Workouts

As the fitness benefits of salsa and other Latin dance forms have become clear, salsa has moved beyond the dance clubs and into gyms and fitness centers across the country and throughout the world. Various kinds of fitness classes crank up the enjoyment factor of exercise by combining dance moves with traditional workout moves.

One of the most popular of these is Zumba, which was created by Alberto Perez, a Colombian dancer, choreographer, and cyclist, in the 1990s. (The official Zumba motto is: "Ditch the workout. Join the party!") Zumba combines moves from a variety of dance styles, such as salsa, hip-hop, merengue, flamenco, soca, and mambo, as well as strength-training moves such as lunges and squats.

What I like so much about Zumba is that it's not just fun — it's actually a fantastic workout. A study by the American Council on Exercise found that doing Zumba burns more than 9 calories a minute, which is about as much as jogging or biking fifteen miles per hour. "It's a total-body exercise — a good, high-energy aerobic workout," said John Porcari, PhD, of the University of Wisconsin–La Crosse's Department of Exercise and Sport Science. "Zumba fitness is also good for core strengthening and flexibility gains because there are lots of hip and midsection movements."

Other research has found that Zumba is a very effective activity for weight loss. For example, researchers found that when overweight and obese women with type 2 diabetes did Zumba three times a week for sixteen weeks, they successfully lost weight as well as body fat. And much to the researchers' delight, many of the women in the study continued attending their Zumba classes even after the study ended. "It seems like most of them had fun, made friends, and didn't see Zumba as hard work," noted study coauthor Jamie Cooper, an associate professor at the University of Georgia.

Zumba seems to appeal to many of the people who don't like typical exercise regimens. I checked out a Zumba class recently at a YMCA, and I saw dozens of people of all ages, all sizes, and all fitness levels dancing and laughing and working up a great sweat. They were having a blast—much more fun than the people on the stationary bikes. But what pleased me even more was learning that several of the Zumba class regulars usually went out for coffee after class. And some of them went out dancing together occasionally at a Latin dance club nearby. What a wonderful way to build friendships as well as fitness!

To find a Zumba class near you, go to www.zumba.com and plug in your zip code.

And Don't Forget Walking

Although I find salsa dancing to be one of the most enjoyable, rewarding activities, I have to put in a plug for walking, because it's one of the easiest, best fitness activities. You can walk anytime, anywhere—all you need is a comfortable pair of shoes, and you've got a workout.

Brisk walking (walking at a pace of three miles an hour or faster) delivers the same health benefits as other activities that get your heart rate into the cardio zone. It's especially good for people who are obese or who have never exercised before, as well as those who feel self-conscious about exercising.

Start with an easy, comfortable pace for the first few minutes of your walk. As you warm up, speed up a bit. Don't worry if you can only walk for a few minutes, or if you walk at a snail's pace. What matters is that you're out there putting one foot in front of the other. If you're new to exercise, plan to walk slowly for five minutes a day every day for a week. Then push up to ten minutes a day. Increase your daily walks gradually, and before you know it, you'll be walking longer and faster. Your goal at the start is to build a fitness habit, not to win races.

As your fitness level increases, you can add challenges to make your walk more of a workout. For example, you can walk faster, farther, or more frequently. You can walk up hills or stairs. You can add occasional bursts of speed to your walks. And you can mix walking and jogging, if you'd like.

Walking is a great activity to do with other people. Instead of meeting a friend for a meal or snack, go for a walk! You'll be amazed at how much distance you can cover while you chat and catch up. And if you're out walking, you won't be eating heavy meals or rich desserts.

For optimal safety, use common sense when you head outdoors. Walk on sidewalks, wear bright-colored clothing, carry a flashlight at night, and keep the volume down if you listen to music or podcasts so you can maintain awareness of what's going on around you.

Break It into Ten-Minute "Bursts"

Unfortunately, despite the many advantages of exercise, only about half of American adults meet the recommended guidelines for cardio activity. And fewer of us—only one in five—meet guidelines for aerobic exercise and muscle strengthening.

Why don't people get the exercise they need? One big factor is time. Guidelines from the Centers for Disease Control and Prevention recommend a total of 150 minutes per week (two and a half hours) of moderate-intensity exercise such as brisk walking, as well as two weekly sessions of muscle-strengthening activities that work all major muscle groups.

I get it—150 minutes sounds like a lot, and I think hearing that number puts off a lot of people. They may feel intimidated by the idea of exercising for two and a half hours each week, and they may engage in all-or-nothing thinking and tell themselves that if they can't meet that goal, there's no point in doing any exercise at all. The truth is, any activity is better than no activity, so even if you can't meet lofty exercise goals, you can still have an impact on your weight and your health.

Here's another important thing you should know about exercise before you write it off with the assumption that you don't have time for it. You probably know people who run for miles a day or swim for an hour every morning. But the fact is that you don't have to schedule big blocks of time for exercise. Many studies have found that spreading out activity into ten-minute chunks throughout the day is as effective as doing longer periods of exercise. You may not have time for half-hour exercise sessions most days of the week, but few of us can truly say that we can't fit a few ten-minute activity "bursts" into our days. It's easy to do a salsa dancing activity burst—play three or four songs, and you're all set. Show your moves, or do it in private—but do it!

Instead of saying you don't have time for exercise because you can't devote a big chunk of time to it each day, try something like this: Go for a ten-minute walk in the morning before work. Turn on music and salsa dance for ten minutes after lunch. Grab your bike when you get home and go for a ten-minute ride around the neighborhood. Or spend ten minutes doing a mini-workout that includes jogging in place, jumping jacks, sit-ups, squats, planks, and triceps dips while you watch television in the evening.

Your goal during these ten-minute activity bursts is to move briskly enough to get your heart beating faster, moving your heart rate into the "cardio zone." What does this mean? Numerically, the target cardio zone heart rate for moderate-intensity activity is anywhere from 100 to 150 beats per minute, depending on your age and your fitness level. If you're a numbers geek, feel free to buy yourself a heart-rate monitor and learn all about using your age and your maximum heart rate to figure out exactly what your target cardio zone heart rate should be. But if you'd rather keep things easy, simply use the talk test to determine whether you're hitting the cardio zone: You know you're doing moderate-intensity cardio zone activity if you can talk, but not sing, while you exercise. As you go along, slow down a little if you can't talk, and speed up if you can easily sing while you exercise. Let Marc Anthony do the singing! You just move those legs, shake those hips, and please, do all of this with your intense salsa look on. Get infected with that Latin passion!

Don't consider these ten-minute exercise sessions as punishments.

Instead, think of them as breaks you take from your day, kind of like coffee breaks—only better. Exercise energizes you in a way that caffeine doesn't. Once you get your heart pumping, you're likely to discover that you have more energy, feel less tired, and are better able to focus on whatever else is on your to-do list each day.

You are more likely to exercise if you truly make it a priority in your life. I had a patient who told me that he wanted to lose weight very badly, but he never made it a priority to change his diet or start exercising—in other words, what he was saying didn't match his actions. He was in the catering business, and his work was very important to him. I once asked him, "Are exercise and weight loss as important to you as your business?" He said yes. Then I asked him, "If that's the case, why don't you put exercise on your calendar as you do with your business meetings and catering activities?" He got my point, and he started to add exercise to his schedule, prioritizing it just as he did with his business commitments. He told me that he took his workouts as seriously as his work, and wouldn't answer the phone while he was exercising, even if the call was from a potential new customer. Within six months, he had lost thirty pounds.

Thinking Strategies to Activate You

In chapter 2 we talked about the process of restructuring negative automatic thoughts about diets and weight loss. This technique is also a useful way to turn around your negative thoughts about exercise. Here are some ways you can redirect your thinking to help you invite more activity into your life.

▸ **HURTFUL NEGATIVE THOUGHT:** I can't exercise because I am too overweight, and my health is too poor.

Helpful restructured thought: Dr. Juan said that exercise is safe for most people, even those who are overweight or obese or who have chronic health problems. Just to be sure, I will check with my doctor. If she says it's safe for me to exercise, I will give it a try. Because I feel worried about it, though, I'll start with something simple, such as a walk around the block, and I'll ask my spouse to accompany me in case I feel unwell along the way.

▸ **HURTFUL NEGATIVE THOUGHT**: I can't exercise because I would be too embarrassed to join an exercise class or go to a gym.

Helpful restructured thought: I can exercise on my own, without going to a class or a gym. I can salsa dance in my home, walk in my neighborhood, or cycle on the bike path by the beach. Maybe someday when I feel more confident I can think about taking an exercise class, but for now I can exercise perfectly well on my own.

▸ **HURTFUL NEGATIVE THOUGHT**: I don't have time to exercise.

Helpful restructured thought: It's true, my schedule is very busy. But if losing weight and improving my health are important to me, I can find the time to exercise. And I don't have to exercise for long periods of time—I can break it up into ten-minute fitness bursts. I'll try different things, such as getting up ten minutes earlier in the morning and going for a walk before work. Also, I'll examine my schedule to see if there are any changes I can make to carve out time for exercise. I do find time to watch television every evening; perhaps I can watch a little less TV to give myself a little more time for exercise. Or I can exercise while I watch TV.

▸ **HURTFUL NEGATIVE THOUGHT**: When I've tried to exercise in the past, I found it boring, so there's no point in trying it again.

Helpful restructured thought: In the past, I tried going to the gym and walking on the treadmill for thirty minutes a day. It really was boring! This time, I'm going to take a new tack. I'm going to try several different activities, such as salsa dancing, hiking outdoors, and asking a friend who loves tennis to teach me how to play. Maybe I'll even think about checking out the adult soccer league my sister belongs to. If I try something and I don't like it, rather than writing off exercise completely, I'll just try something else.

▶ **HURTFUL NEGATIVE THOUGHT**: I'm too tired to exercise.

Helpful restructured thought: Yes, I'm exhausted when I get home from work. But I'm not so tired at other times of the day, so I will exercise during those times when I feel more energetic, such as in the morning, during my lunch break, and on days off from work. Also, Dr. Juan says that activity can be invigorating, so I'm going to experiment with doing ten minutes of exercise after work and see how I feel. Maybe it will help energize me after a long day at work!

▶ **HURTFUL NEGATIVE THOUGHT**: There's no way I can exercise for the recommended 150 minutes a week, so I'm not going to bother doing anything.

Helpful restructured thought: Having this all-or-nothing view on exercise isn't helpful to me. Any amount of exercise is beneficial, even if I can't hit the 150 minutes per week mark. I will start small, with 10 minutes of exercise a day. Then, after I build that habit into my day, I will add another 10 minutes a day.

Here's another way to think about exercise: not as a chore you must add to your to-do list or a requirement foisted on you by your doctor, but as a gift that you give yourself as a reward for the hard work you do for yourself, your employer, and your family. We all deserve to take time for ourselves—time to take care of ourselves. If you really can't carve out a few ten-minute breaks for yourself each day, perhaps you have too much going on. It's worth asking yourself whether there are changes you should consider making, such as asking your partner to take on more housework or childcare, or talking with your boss about balancing your workload. We all need time to take care of ourselves.

MOJITO DIET SUCCESS STORY: VANESSA

Reversing the Medical Family History

Vanessa's family health history played a big part in her decision to follow the Mojito Diet. "I have many family members with high blood pressure, high cholesterol, and high blood sugar," says Vanessa, forty, who works as an office administrator. "When I saw my cholesterol numbers increasing, I knew it was time to take action. I wanted to lower my cholesterol naturally before having to consider taking medication."

During her first twelve weeks on the Mojito Diet, Vanessa saw some very impressive results: She lost twenty pounds, and her waist measurement decreased by three inches. But perhaps even more exciting was the dramatic improvement in her cholesterol levels. Vanessa's LDL, or "bad" cholesterol, dropped from 155 to 83, and her total cholesterol fell from 219 to 167.

In the past, Vanessa had tried weight-loss programs that delivered ready-to-eat foods to her home. Although she enjoyed having her meals prepared for her, the programs weren't as helpful as she would have hoped. "The food delivery got expensive, and I still had to cook all the meals for my family. And they didn't include a plan for when you stop the meals."

With the Mojito Diet, Vanessa prepares healthy meals that fit her weight-loss plan and satisfy her family. "Being able to cook the same thing for the whole family is the best. Everyone serves themselves as usual, and I serve myself the right-size portions. I am a good role model for my children, and now I am a role model for healthy eating at home."

Vanessa appreciates having an easy way to track the types of fats she eats, and she looks forward to her end-of-the-week mojitos. "Having them guilt-free makes them taste that much better. Following a diet that rewards you with a yummy mojito is superb," Vanessa says. And, to top it all off, Vanessa says that now that she makes Mojito Water, not only does she drink more water every day, but her skin has cleared up too.

"This is a lifestyle change for the better," Vanessa says. "You learn to make good-tasting healthy food at home, and you learn how to make smart and healthy choices on the days you dine out. I'm psyched about the Mojito Diet—I am sticking to it!"

5

~~~

Set Yourself Up for Success

We've talked about a lot of important topics so far—why weight loss matters, how to reframe automatic negative thoughts about weight loss, using rewards to keep you motivated, and making fitness fun. Now, before we dig in deep on what you'll be eating as you follow the Mojito Diet, let's look at a few other strategies that can pave the way to effective weight loss.

Document your before and after

Some people like to document their "before" status by photographing themselves and taking various body measurements. If you think this will help you, go ahead and do it—but if it will make you feel bad about yourself, don't bother.

Prepare your kitchen

Some diet books ask you to throw away every food in your kitchen that doesn't fit exactly into their plan. You don't have to do that with the Mojito Diet because my plan doesn't forbid you to eat any foods. Yes, I will ask you to fill your plate with many healthy foods, and to limit certain foods that can interfere with weight loss. But I won't tell you that you can never eat this or that, because if you're anything like me, that will just make you want those foods more! (Hmmm. Maybe if I tell you never to eat kale, you'll start to crave it.)

Rather than expecting you to rent a Dumpster to cart away every snack chip, cookie, and sweet in your house, I'll only ask you to look around your kitchen and think about whether you'd be better off without certain foods that easily cause you to overeat—let's call them "trigger foods." For me, desserts are trigger foods—especially desserts like the coconut cheese flan my wife sometimes makes for special occasions like Thanksgiving. It's a recipe from her father's restaurant, and it is, in my opinion, the best flan on earth. When that flan is in my house, I can't stop thinking about it (or eating it!). I rarely ask my wife to make it, because I know I can't be trusted with it. If I were starting a diet, I would make sure there was none of that flan in my kitchen!

For the snack foods that remain, consider rearranging your cabinets and drawers to put them out of sight. Sometimes just seeing a food makes you want it, so you're better off not being able to lay eyes on it.

As you prepare your kitchen, check to see if you have measuring cups, measuring spoons, and a food scale for checking portion sizes. You won't always have to measure your food, but I do recommend it at first, because most of us are terrible at guessing portion sizes. You'll also want to make sure you have the appropriate containers for packing lunches and storing leftovers. I think you'll enjoy the recipes in this book so much that you'll want to double them so there's plenty left over for lunch the next day or freezing for another meal in the future. Finally, pull out a big bowl for fruit, because it's an important part of the Mojito Diet.

Go grocery shopping

As you start following the Mojito Diet, you might need to make some changes to your usual grocery shopping habits. For example, the Mojito Diet may include more vegetables and fruit than you're accustomed to eating. And some of the recipes I've included in each week of meal plans call for foods or spices you may not have on hand. (Spices are an important ingredient in my recipes, so make sure your spice rack is full!) However, I won't be asking you to buy foods that require trips to stores all over town—generally, everything you need should be available in your usual supermarket.

Enlist support

It's great to have friends, family members, neighbors, and coworkers support you as you set out on your weight-loss journey.

Start by trying to get buy-in from your immediate family. Explain why you want to lose weight, what changes you'll be making to your diet, and how you may be changing your schedule to make room for physical activity. Invite them to be part of your journey, but don't take it personally if they aren't interested in jumping on the Mojito Diet bandwagon with you. We all have to come to weight loss and healthy eating when we are ready, and it will only backfire if you try to force your spouse or other family members to make changes if they don't want to.

If you do most of the cooking and meal preparation in your house, work with your family to create a strategy that will allow you to follow your healthy eating plans without having to prepare two sets of meals—I bet that when they taste my Mojito Diet recipes, they'll want to eat what you're having even if they're not trying to lose weight.

Think about who in your life might be willing to support you, and talk with them about exactly what they can do to contribute to your efforts. For example, ask your mother to take care of your kids on Saturday mornings so you can go to your Zumba class, make a plan with your dog-walking neighbor to accompany her on her evening strolls, or ask your spouse to help with grocery shopping or cutting up fruits and vegetables for meals. Look for people who might want to partner with you on your quest and help keep you accountable; like so many other things in life, weight loss is easier when you're doing it with someone else.

When you tell family and friends that you're starting a weight-loss program, you'll probably get lots of support. But don't be surprised if you get some blowback too.

Spouses, family members, and friends occasionally feel threatened when someone they love starts to eat better or exercise more. Some of the people in your life won't support the changes you're making; in fact, they may actively try to sabotage you by tempting you with your favorite treats, suggesting that you skip your workouts, or bad-mouthing your healthy choices.

If this happens, try talking with those people in a kind, loving way. Recognize that change can be threatening for some people—even when it's positive—and acknowledge that they may feel guilty about their own choices or envious of you for having the motivation to try to make improvements in your health. But stand firm in your commitment to pursue eating and activity goals that will help you lose weight and improve your health.

If you can't win their support, seek it elsewhere, from friends or family members who can cheer you on happily and without their own issues getting in the way. Ultimately, we must all make our own decisions about our health.

Start a food and fitness diary

I recommend keeping a food and fitness diary for three very important reasons.

First, it encourages you to pay attention to what you're eating and doing in a way that you are less likely to do when you're not writing it down.

Second, it helps keep you honest—you're less likely to fudge on serving sizes or food choices when you've promised yourself to record everything you're eating in your food diary.

And third, research has found that people who maintain food and fitness diaries are more successful at weight loss than those who skip this important step. In fact, one study of 1,700 people found that those who tracked their food intake lost twice as much weight as those who didn't. That's a significant benefit from an action that takes only a couple of minutes each day.

We are inclined to underestimate how much we eat and overestimate how much we move. But keeping track of it and writing it down pushes you to be more mindful about your choices and their impact on you. Having a record of your daily eating and exercise can teach you a lot about yourself—for example, you may not realize how much or how often you eat, or how little you exercise. You may even want to begin tracking what you eat and do *before* you start following the Mojito Diet, so that you can clearly see the differences in your before-and-after choices.

When you start your food and fitness diary, use whatever format suits you best, either paper or electronic. For food, write down what you eat and drink for each meal and snack, along with the amount of food, what time you ate, where you ate, and how you felt before and after eating. If you're not exactly sure how much you ate, make an estimate, but do so as accurately as possible. Even if you ate too much, or chose foods that you hadn't planned on having, write it all down. Tell yourself the truth about snacks you sneaked or the amount of food you ate—nobody has to see it but you. Cheating on what you report in your food and fitness diary won't do you any favors.

Once a week or so, go back to your food and fitness diary and look for trends. Having an accurate record to examine can help you recognize times, foods, or moods that are linked to overeating or habits that may need changing or successes that are worth repeating. You can identify and recognize situations that lead to overeating or skipping exercise, as well as circumstances that enabled success. For example, your food diary may tell you that you tend to overeat when you socialize with a certain friend, or that you do kick-ass workouts in the mornings but not the evenings. Use whatever trends you notice to fine-tune your eating and activity plans going forward.

You don't have to keep a food and fitness diary forever, although if it's helping, you may want to stick with it. But as you set out on your weight-loss journey, it's incredibly helpful to have an honest, detailed reckoning of exactly what you're doing and not doing. That way, you can make the adjustments necessary to help you meet your goals.

Gear up for exercise

Don't worry—I'm not going to tell you to spend thousands of dollars on a treadmill or hundreds on designer gym wear. But I would like you to invest a small amount of money in a good pair of athletic shoes and whatever else you may need to be safe, supported, and comfortable while you're physically active. You are far more likely to stick to your workout plan if you feel comfortable while you're doing it.

For walking and salsa dancing, all you need is a decent pair of sneakers with cushioning and arch support. No need to spend a lot on shoes—as long as you're not particular about brands and colors, you can get what you need on sale or at a discount store. Make sure your sneakers fit properly—snug but not tight, with enough room to wiggle your toes. Shoe experts suggest shopping for sneakers later in the day, because your feet tend to swell slightly as the day goes on. Buy them first thing in the morning and you may discover they don't fit as well in the evening.

In addition to shoes, you may want to buy a few pairs of socks designed for physical activity, if you need them. Pick socks that fit well, to protect you from blisters. Choose plain cotton or synthetic fabrics that wick sweat away from your skin. Cushioned socks are nice, but not necessary unless you would benefit from the extra support they provide.

As for clothing, there's no reason to go out and buy all the latest workout fashions—unless you want to, of course. If having new exercise clothes motivates you, go ahead and replenish your wardrobe, or buy yourself something new as a reward for meeting a performance goal. But if the thought of going to a sporting goods store and trying on activewear makes you sweat, skip it.

DR. JUAN'S WISDOM

STRAP ON A STEP COUNTER

Although it's not necessary, a step counter such as a Fitbit or a step-counting smartphone app is a nice way to track your activity for the day, especially if you're a numbers geek. Some of my patients find they are much more active when they set a daily goal of, say, ten thousand steps a day and track their progress on their step counter.

I have a patient who literally will not go to bed until she hits the ten-thousand-step mark. If she's short for the day, she will pace around the house and walk up and down the stairs before bedtime to get the steps she needs to make the fireworks on her Fitbit go off.

You can also monitor your progress by writing down how many minutes you're active. But if a step tracker will help keep you motivated and you can afford it, consider purchasing one.

Get enough sleep

Believe it or not, sleep and weight are connected in important ways. Some are pretty obvious—when you're tired, it's tough to summon the energy for physical activity, and it's common to turn to food to perk you up when you're feeling worn out and lethargic. And who feels like cooking a healthy dinner when they're exhausted? Being chronically tired really can compromise your ability to make good decisions for your health.

There's more to it than that, though. Research has shown that when we're tired, we're more likely to crave high-fat, high-carbohydrate foods, especially sweet-salty snack foods. That's because tiredness messes with the brain's ability to control our desires. Lack of sleep also interferes with the action of hormones such as leptin, ghrelin, and cortisol, which play a part in appetite, hunger, and fullness. If you're not getting enough rest, you may want to make sleep more of a priority as you start the Mojito Diet.

How much sleep do you need? Although it varies by individual, most of us feel the most refreshed and productive with seven to nine hours of sleep per night. To determine exactly how much you need, ask yourself a few questions: Do you feel sleepy during the day? Do you need frequent jolts of caffeine to keep yourself going? Do you struggle to stay awake while watching movies, sitting in meetings, or driving? If so, you probably need more sleep than you're getting. To keep track of how much sleep you're getting, consider including daily hours of sleep in your food and fitness diary.

Some simple steps can help you get better sleep. Stick to a schedule, make your bedroom sleep-friendly (cool, dark, and quiet), avoid looking at electronic devices close to bedtime, and stay away from caffeine and alcohol in the evenings if they interfere with your sleep. For me, creating a bedtime routine was very helpful. For many years I suffered from insomnia and was sleeping an average of only five hours per night. It wasn't until I changed my sleep hygiene that I started getting my eight hours in. I have a routine: I drink a passion fruit tea before going to bed, advice I got from a shaman I met in Guatemala when I was recording my TV show *Strange Medicine*. I don't bring the computer or any type of work to my bed. My phone is on my night table because I have no choice—I am a concierge physician, so I'm always on call. But I don't use it during that time to check e-mails or browse the Web. And I don't watch the news! Instead, I look at the same TV show every night: *Seinfeld*. It is a show I love and it makes me laugh even though I know each episode by heart. My brain knows that when *Seinfeld* comes on, it's time for bed—and in about fifteen minutes, I am usually asleep.

DR. JUAN'S WISDOM

SPEAK UP IF YOU CAN'T SLEEP

Good sleep isn't a luxury—you need it for optimal health and successful weight loss.

Some sleep problems have a medical cause. Talk with your doctor if you find yourself waking up often, if you experience morning headaches or dry mouth, or if your sleep partner notices that you're waking up frequently, snoring, gasping, or choking during the night. These can be signs of obstructive sleep apnea, a common sleep disorder that is prevalent among overweight and obese people. Sleep apnea and other sleep disorders can be successfully treated, so be sure to tell your doctor if you're having trouble getting the rest you need.

Sleep quality can also suffer in women experiencing nighttime hot flashes; sometimes treatments such as hormone therapy or low-dose antidepressants can help.

Address stress

Like sleep, stress plays an important part in your ability to lose weight. When you're stressed, your body produces stress hormones such as cortisol, known as the "fight or flight" hormone, which gives your body the boost it needs to deal with dangerous situations. Once danger passes, your cortisol level returns to normal. However, if you face chronic stress over an extended period—for example, a boss who treats you badly on a regular basis, money problems that worry you every day, or a family member facing a serious health crisis—your cortisol levels may remain elevated for long periods of time.

Chronic stress and excess cortisol affect your body in many ways. For example, they can prevent you from getting a good night's sleep, raise your blood pressure, and interfere with your insulin/blood sugar levels, causing you to crave carbohydrates. Excess cortisol from chronic stress can also contribute to the storage of extra fat around your middle and deep within your belly. This "visceral fat," as it's known, releases chemicals that contribute to inflammation that raises the risk of health conditions such as diabetes and heart disease. Chronically high levels of stress hormones also slow down your metabolism, which makes it harder for you to burn off calories from food and lose weight.

Nonstop stress can make it harder for you to stay committed to your weight-loss plan. When you're stressed, you're less likely to make healthy choices about food and exercise. I'm sure you've heard the term *stress eating*. For many of us, food is a go-to when we feel stressed. Gobbling up a stack of cookies or a pint of ice cream may feel relaxing as you eat, but as soon as you finish, you are likely to feel even more stressed because you've eaten so much. And, even though we know exercise helps reduce stressful feelings, you may be tempted to skip your workouts when stress levels soar.

Sometimes we can eliminate the stressors in our lives. For example, if your drive to work through horrible rush-hour traffic causes you major stress, you may be able to commute by train or bus instead. But often our stressors are beyond our control—quitting a job to get away from an annoying boss, say, simply may not be an option. That's where stress-relief techniques and relaxation strategies come in.

When we take steps to relax our bodies, we give ourselves a break from the stressors in our lives. Relaxation strategies such as meditation, yoga, deep breathing, mindfulness, visualization, journaling, spending enjoyable time with people we like, receiving social support from others, and exercise are just some of the tools we can use to relax ourselves and give our bodies a break from chronic stress. Engaging in stress-reduction techniques like these can actually lower the levels of cortisol in your blood. Even taking a few minutes to think about the things in your life for which you are thankful can give you a break from stress.

If you've got major chronic stress in your life, I urge you to make whatever changes possible to alleviate it. And to help you cope with the stressors you can't change, I hope that you'll try some of these relaxation techniques to identify coping strategies that work for you. Doing so will help you reduce the effect of chronic stress on your health—and help you meet your diet, exercise, and weight-loss goals.

MOJITO DIET SUCCESS STORY: **DENY**

After Trying Every Single Diet

Around the time she turned forty, Deny started to gain weight. This is a common problem for women in their forties and fifties: Even though they aren't necessarily eating more or moving less than they had in the past, their weight just starts to creep up. It's a very frustrating situation caused by hormonal shifts, a loss of muscle mass, and an increase in body fat.

"I tried so many different diets, and nothing seemed to work," says Deny, forty-seven, a sonographer. "I tried the no-carbs diet, and it was so hard to do that I eventually quit. I also tried counting calories, and that was very difficult, too, because I always needed to be keeping track of every calorie I ate."

Everything changed for Deny when she started to follow the Mojito Diet. Within days, Deny began to see changes on the scale and in her body even though she wasn't counting calories or eliminating all carbs. Finally, she found a plan that worked for her. In just sixteen weeks, Deny lost twenty-two pounds.

Deny isn't just thrilled about her weight loss, but about improving the quality of her diet. Working in a medical office, she knows firsthand what an unhealthy diet can do. "I finally learned to eat healthy meals with food from all food groups," Deny says. "I'm more cautious about the types of food I eat and the serving sizes. This is now a way of life for me, and I couldn't be happier. I'm eating healthier, I have more energy, and I feel great."

The weight-loss plans Deny had tried before the Mojito Diet focused on what she *couldn't* eat, so she was happy to follow a plan that allowed so many of her favorite foods, including alcohol. "I enjoy that I am able to eat all types of food in each food group, and still lose weight. And the best part is that I am able to enjoy an occasional glass of wine, without any guilt!"

PART TWO

GET READY TO EAT AND DRINK

In part 1 of this book we looked at some of the ways in which you can achieve weight-loss success by changing the way you think about diet and exercise. In this section, we're going to talk about the specific food choices that can fuel your weight loss.

We'll start with protein and carbohydrates. Protein is the engine that drives weight loss, but carbohydrates are also a crucial part of the equation. So many eating plans eliminate or sharply cut down on carbohydrates, but the Mojito Diet puts them back on the table because of the critical role they play.

We'll also talk about sixteen-hour fasting, a surprisingly simple, effective way to eat less and lose more. And I'll tell you how the delicious foods included in the Mojito Diet can help protect your heart and your brain from the chronic diseases that can steal joy from your life.

Along the way, I'll share lots of fantastic tips for making smart eating choices that will help you meet your goals while enjoying every meal you eat.

The Mojito Diet brings together a range of best practices that can pave the way to successful long-term weight loss and optimal health.

6

Put Protein to
Work for You

There's something about protein that seems to strike a deep emotional
chord in so many of us. Perhaps it's because meat, seafood, cheese, milk,
and other protein foods are so tied up with our memories from childhood.
For example, when I was a kid in Puerto Rico, we feasted on *lechón*, a
whole spit-roasted pig, on Christmas Eve. Protein was part of all sorts of
other circumstances too. Homemade chicken soup to soothe a sore throat.
A grill full of hamburgers to kick off summer. A big pot of *bacalao* (fish
stew) for Sunday night suppers. And of course, my mother's grilled cheese
sandwiches with a mug of tomato soup to ease the pain of a disappointment. Protein is our go-to food for celebration, anguish, and comfort,
providing us with solid sustenance that is emotional as well as physical.

Protein comes through for us when we're facing the challenge of losing
weight too. Many studies have found that including a healthy amount of
protein in our diets can help with weight loss and weight maintenance
by increasing feelings of fullness after eating and fending off hunger and
food cravings between meals.

The trick, of course, is to eat the right amount of protein, and the right
kinds of protein foods. Sometimes when we think a food is going to help
us lose weight, we go overboard with it, thinking that if some is good,
more must be better. Protein is most effective for weight loss when you're
including some at each meal and snack, as you will when you follow the
Mojito Diet, and choosing protein foods that provide the most bang for

your nutritional buck. But too much protein—or the wrong kinds—can interfere with weight loss and health.

In this chapter we'll take a good look at how protein helps with weight loss, which types of protein provide the best nutritional benefits, and the optimal amount of protein to eat for weight loss and overall health. And while we're at it, we'll talk a little about dietary fat too.

Feel Full Longer

Have you ever noticed that sometimes, only a short time after eating, you feel hungry again? And other times, you go for hours without thinking about food? A big reason for the discrepancy in how long it takes to feel hungry again after eating is the amount of protein in the meal. Protein does a great job of making you feel satiated—in fact, researchers believe that protein is better at leaving you feeling satisfied after a meal than fat or carbohydrates.

To determine this, researchers do experiments that go something like this: They give half of a group of study subjects a high-protein meal, and the other half a low-protein meal. Then they ask the study subjects to rate how hungry they feel during the hours after they've eaten their meals. Overall, study subjects who eat high-protein meals say they feel fuller for a longer time than those who eat low-protein meals.

Some studies add a further twist: When it's time for another meal, researchers invite the subjects from both groups to help themselves to a meal from a buffet. Subjects are not told how much to eat—they simply eat what they are hungry for. After the study participants finish, the researchers measure how much they've eaten. Inevitably, researchers find that the participants who had eaten the high-protein meals earlier tend to have eaten less at the buffet meal than those who had eaten the low-protein meals earlier in the day. This suggests that even if you're not actively trying to drop pounds, eating protein at each meal and snack could help you lose weight (or avoid gaining it). So imagine how helpful protein is when you're following a plan like the Mojito Diet that is designed to help you trim down!

Why would a protein-rich meal help you feel more satiated? There are a few reasons. One has to do with the hormones leptin (which *decreases* hunger) and ghrelin (which *increases* hunger). When you eat protein, your body releases less ghrelin (the "hunger hormone") and more leptin (the "satiety hormone") than it does when you eat carbohydrates or fat.

Researchers found proof of this when they fed one group of volunteers a high-protein breakfast and the other a low-protein breakfast. When the researchers measured the amount of ghrelin in the volunteers' bodies a few hours later, they found that those who had eaten the high-protein breakfast had less ghrelin in their blood than those who ate the low-protein breakfast.

If those aren't enough reasons to make sure to include lean protein in each meal and snack, as we do in the Mojito Diet, here are a couple more:

Protein prevents blood sugar spikes

Eating a meal that contains lots of low-quality carbohydrates from refined grains and sugars causes your blood sugar to shoot up rapidly. When it falls, it triggers hunger pangs that send you searching for more food. I am very familiar with this kind of sugar rush. As a matter of fact, I consider myself a recovering sugar addict. I love desserts! I grew up with desserts being an important part of almost every meal. We enjoyed them as a family, and my mother loved making them for us. And, as I mentioned earlier, as an adult I have been known to pick a restaurant based on the desserts they serve! Flan and *tres leches* drive me nuts. But I have learned how to combat these urges by carefully regulating the amount of lean protein that I eat.

When you eat a meal that contains protein, your blood sugar goes up and comes down more slowly, and you avoid the rapid blood sugar drop that makes your stomach growl with hunger soon after eating. Instead, because protein slows down digestion and the absorption of sugar into your blood, you feel more satiated and less hungry for a longer amount of time.

Protein feeds muscle

Protein is a favorite fuel for muscle tissue. If you don't get enough of it when you're losing weight, you risk losing muscle as well as fat. You can preserve and build your muscles by exercising, strength training, and eating lean protein. Studies have found that people on higher-protein weight-loss diets preserve and gain more muscle than those on low-protein diets, especially if they include strength-building exercise in their regular routines.

Protein burns calories

This is one of my favorite benefits that protein brings to the table: Digesting proteins actually uses up more energy—that is, calories—than digesting other kinds of food. When you eat a meal or snack, your body has to break it down in order to use it for energy. Because of the way protein molecules are designed, protein is more difficult to break down than fat or carbohydrates. In fact, as much as 20 to 30 percent of the calories in protein is used up by the protein digestion process, compared with less than 10 percent for carbs and 3 percent for fat.

To put it very simply, when you eat 100 calories of lean protein, only 70 to 80 of them "count" in the final calorie tally for that food. What's more, because protein digestion is a greater effort for your body, it revs up your metabolism throughout the day (and night). That's a pretty great payoff, as far as I'm concerned.

Making Smart Protein Choices

Although protein helps with weight loss in a variety of ways, eating excessive amounts of it can backfire on you. Too much protein can be harmful to your bones, kidneys, and liver. And if most of your protein is coming from red meat and processed meats, it could increase your risk of colorectal cancer and heart disease. Following the Mojito Diet should take you to your protein sweet spot—enough for weight loss, but not enough to raise health risks.

One of the best ways to optimize protein's power is to eat protein-rich foods that provide more than just protein. For example, when you drink milk, you're getting a healthy dose of calcium and vitamin D in addition to protein. Beans, seeds, and nuts provide fiber as well as protein. And plant-based protein offers antioxidants and a wealth of other nutrients too.

Now that we've looked at how protein can help you with weight loss and health, let's talk about which protein-rich foods you'll be including in the meals and snacks you eat as you follow the Mojito Diet.

Lean Meats: Make Mine Sirloin

When I talk about high-protein food, meat is probably the first food that enters your mind—especially the red meats (beef, lamb, and pork—despite what the advertisements say, pork is a "red" meat, not a "white" meat like poultry), as well as processed meat (sausage, bacon, hot dogs, and luncheon meat). Red meat and processed meats do provide protein, but I can't recommend that you eat them frequently or in large quantities, as some very low-carbohydrate, very high-protein diets do. Limited amounts of lean meat are fine—it's included in the Mojito Diet—but eating too much meat, or choosing fatty meat, does have drawbacks. And it's best to limit processed meats because of their links to cancer.

Let's start with lean versus fatty meat. Although the Mojito Diet doesn't focus heavily on calories, it does limit the number of calories you eat each day. Calories matter for weight loss, and eating too many of them leads to weight gain. Fatty meat is much higher in calories than lean meat, so it's best for your weight to choose lean cuts and to remove as much visible fat as you can manage. And it's best to avoid lard (pork fat), which is commonly used in some Latin recipes.

I also recommend limiting meat because of its potential impact on heart health. There's a large body of evidence linking meat to heart disease. For example, a well-respected twenty-eight-year study of 120,000 people conducted by Harvard researchers found that people who ate the most red meat were more likely to die younger, and had higher rates of heart disease and cancer, than those who ate the least red meat. Risk of early death and disease were highest among people who ate the most processed meat, such as bacon, hot dogs, and cold cuts.

In another very large study, researchers at the National Cancer Institute looked at the meat-eating habits of 537,000 people over age fifty for sixteen years. They found that eating red meat (processed and unprocessed) was associated with death due to nine different causes, including cancer, heart disease, stroke, diabetes, and Alzheimer's disease.

You may argue that studies like these show association, not causation — in other words, they do not definitively prove that red meat and processed meat are what caused health problems and earlier death in the study subjects. You may wonder whether other factors may have played a role in illness or death — for example, maybe the people in these studies who ate large amounts of red meat also smoked cigarettes or drank too much alcohol or didn't exercise. And studying people's eating patterns over long periods of time, especially when researchers depend on their subjects to remember and write down what they've eaten for months, years, or decades, can be very challenging. Well, it's true that studying people's long-term food choices can be tricky, although researchers do their best to allow for all these factors and challenges and to analyze the data in a way that accounts for them. For example, they typically ask people about their other lifestyle choices and adjust their results accordingly. Despite these qualms, and because these kinds of studies look at such large numbers of people over such long periods of time, I am inclined to take their findings seriously and to recommend that you limit red meat.

Red meat — and fatty red meat in particular — contains saturated fats, which can raise the cholesterol levels in your blood — especially LDL, or "bad" cholesterol. Having high LDL is linked with a higher risk of stroke and heart disease.

Some fad diets allow large amounts of red meat and saturated fat, claiming that it is okay for your heart. But I've seen enough research linking red meat and saturated fat to heart disease that I continue to recommend that we limit our consumption of it, as does the American Heart Association.

I believe in limiting red meat and saturated fat as much as possible. It's much better for your heart to replace some of these foods in your diet with healthier choices like poultry and seafood, as well as nutrient-dense plant-based proteins, including legumes and nuts.

When you do eat meat, try to choose the leanest types of meat and remove all visible fat. The names of meat cuts can vary across the country and in different stores, but lean cuts generally include the words *round*, *sirloin*, or *loin* in their names. The following tend to be the leanest choices:

- Beef: eye of round, top sirloin, flank steak, top round, bottom round, sirloin tip, tenderloin, and lean ground beef (93 percent or higher). "Choice" and "select" grades are leaner than "prime."

- Pork: pork tenderloin, boneless top loin chop, and top loin roast.

- Lamb: loin chop, shank, and boneless leg.

- Other lean meats: lean veal, lean cuts of emu, buffalo, venison, and rabbit. Ham and Canadian bacon are also lean, but tend to be high in sodium.

Healthier Meats?

You may have heard that grass-fed meat is healthier than meat from animals that are fed with conventional grain feed. In fact, there are nutrition experts who believe that research studies like the ones I mentioned have found negative health benefits from red meat because their subjects ate meat from animals fed with grain rather than grass, and that if those same studies were repeated with grass-fed meat they would come out differently. Maybe so — some research does suggest that meat from grass-fed animals is healthier than meat from grain-fed animals. For example, studies have found that grass-fed beef can contain less fat, fewer calories, and higher levels of beneficial antioxidants and omega-3 fatty acids than grain-fed beef.

There are also growing numbers of people who believe that meat is healthier when it comes from animals that are raised organically, allowed to roam free rather than being penned up, protected from exposure to pesticides and fertilizers, and not given antibiotics, growth hormones, or genetically engineered food. It may be that these meats are healthier—but we don't know that for sure, and large-scale studies are a long way off. Meanwhile, organic and grass-fed meat is much more expensive than conventionally raised meat. If you want to buy these varieties and they fit into your grocery budget, go ahead. But if you can't afford them, don't beat yourself up over eating conventionally raised meat.

Instead of getting stressed about paying for grass-fed meat, I'd rather you limit your red meat intake, eat processed meat only occasionally, and choose healthier (and, in some cases, much less expensive) sources of protein, as you will when you follow the Mojito Diet.

As for the diet "experts" who claim that we can eat as much red meat and fatty meat as we'd like without any negative impact on our health and our hearts? I don't believe them. There's too much research pointing in the other direction. As my *abuela* used to say, "If it sounds too good to be true, it probably isn't true."

Poultry

You'll find plenty of poultry in the Mojito Diet. Chicken and turkey provide lots of high-quality protein and are a healthier choice than red meat and processed meat. I recommend removing the skin, because it contains saturated fat and is high in calories. If you choose ground poultry, be sure to choose lean varieties that contain mostly white meat and no skin.

Seafood

The Mojito Diet includes fish and shellfish because they are delicious, nutritious sources of protein that are good for weight loss and your heart. Many types of seafood provide omega-3 fatty acids, which are "good" fats that help your body in a variety of ways.

Let's start with heart health: Omega-3 fatty acids lower the risk of heart arrhythmia, help slow down the accumulation of atherosclerotic plaque, lower triglycerides in the blood, and can help reduce blood pressure. The American Heart Association is so hooked on omega-3-rich fatty fish that it recommends two servings a week, especially if you're at high risk for heart disease. Some of the best choices for your heart are salmon, lake trout, sardines, mackerel, herring, and albacore tuna. (Talk with your doctor before taking fish oil supplements, which are sometimes recommended for people with or at high risk for coronary artery disease.)

The omega-3 fatty acids in seafood help reduce inflammation throughout your body. Some inflammation is fine—it's a normal process that helps your body fight infection. But too much inflammation can be harmful to you, causing damage to your arteries and raising your risk of heart disease, stroke, and type 2 diabetes, as well as other diseases. Chronic inflammation can be caused by a variety of factors, including high blood pressure, obesity, smoking, and stress. Eating seafood helps cool down inflammation, although it's important to take other inflammation-lowering steps also, such as avoiding smoking, reducing stress, and losing weight.

Dairy

You may have seen reports about celebrities endorsing dairy-free diets for weight loss. Their stories sound great: They cut out all dairy and magically drop the stubborn pounds they haven't been able to lose in any other way. Listening to these tales, you may be tempted to eliminate milk, cheese, yogurt, and other dairy from your diet, but I really wouldn't recommend it.

Look at it this way: You'll lose weight if you cut *any* food group out of your daily meal plan and don't replace it with something else. But it's very difficult to sustain this kind of eating for a long period of time, and I can promise you, cutting out all dairy is unlikely to be as effortless as celebrities make it sound. It's also not healthy for you, because dairy foods contain nutrients that your body needs, such as protein, calcium, vitamin D, potassium, and vitamin A.

I include dairy in the Mojito Diet for several reasons. Not only is dairy an excellent source of nutrients, but studies have linked dairy intake to successful weight loss when it's included in diets that cut back on calories. Dairy is a rich source of calcium, which has been linked to weight loss. It's also important for heart health, and is a strategic component of the blood pressure–lowering DASH eating plan, which we'll discuss more in chapter 9. I recommend including at least two servings of dairy in your daily protein intake.

One of my favorite dairy products is yogurt, which delivers not only protein, calcium, and other significant nutrients, but also beneficial bacteria that can have a positive impact on gut health and overall health. These "probiotics" may help lower the risk of digestive problems such as diarrhea, inflammatory bowel disease, and perhaps even cancer of the stomach and colon. Yogurt is an excellent grab-and-go food for breakfast, lunch, or a snack, and it makes a perfect base for smoothies. Be sure to choose plain nonfat yogurt without added sugar, sweetened fruit, candy, or cookies. Add your own fresh fruit and a sprinkle of unsweetened whole-grain granola for a quick, nutritious snack or meal.

There are some types of dairy foods I do suggest you limit or avoid: butter and cream. Both contain substantial amounts of saturated fat, which is linked to heart disease. A small amount occasionally is okay, but in general I recommend using heart-healthy olive oil instead of butter or lard, and having cream (or half-and-half) infrequently. If you're accustomed to pouring it in your coffee, consider switching to milk or drinking your coffee black. At first, coffee without sugar or milk may taste too strong or bitter, but give your taste buds some time to adjust, and you may discover you like the flavor more than you might expect.

Eggs

Good news! We can eat eggs again! For many years, nutrition researchers believed eggs were harmful to heart health because they contain cholesterol. However, it turns out that the cholesterol in eggs doesn't really contribute much to blood cholesterol levels. In fact, eggs may even contribute to heart health by raising "good" HDL cholesterol and lowering stroke risk.

Eggs contain so much good nutrition—not just protein, but vitamin D, vitamin E, several B vitamins, antioxidants such as zeaxanthin and lutein, and choline, which supports brain health, memory, mood, and muscles. And if the eggs you buy are from chickens fed with flaxseed or other omega-3-rich chicken-feed, they may also provide omega-3 fatty acids. Eggs are great for breakfast, of course, but they're also enjoyable in salads or as a snack.

Beans, peas, and lentils

Packed with protein, these tasty little foods are a healthy, economical substitute for meat. They provide plenty of fiber as well as a variety of vitamins and minerals, including iron, B vitamins, calcium, potassium, and more. We'll talk about fiber in chapter 7, but I can tell you right now that most Americans don't get nearly enough fiber. If you start adding more beans, peas, and lentils to your meals, however, you'll be much more likely to hit your healthy fiber targets. Because they contain protein and fiber, these are some of the most filling foods you can find—tuck them into your meal and you're likely to feel full for hours.

Traditional Latin cooking includes lots of beans, peas, and lentils, and they play an important role in the Mojito Diet as well. When you prepare them, you're welcome to make them from scratch. But keep in mind that canned varieties are just as nutritious and can save you a lot of time in the kitchen. Just be sure to drain them and rinse them well before using, to wash off any added salt.

Nuts, nut butters, and seeds

I really can't say enough good things about nuts, nut butters, and seeds. Like beans, peas, and lentils, nuts and seeds are stuffed with fiber and protein. They also contain heart-healthy fat, as well as a range of different nutrients, including vitamins, minerals, and antioxidants. I am always encouraging my patients to include nuts in their diets.

Studies have found that eating nuts on a regular basis is associated with better heart health. For example, in a 2017 study of 210,000 doctors and nurses who reported their diet choices over a period of thirty-two years, researchers found that those people who had nuts five or more times per week saw up to a 20 percent lower risk of heart and artery disease compared with those who never or rarely ate nuts. Other studies have found as much as a 50 percent reduction in the risk of various kinds of heart problems. Evidence in favor of nuts for heart health is so strong that eating an ounce of nuts daily has become standard medical advice.

Because of their protein, fiber, and fat, nuts leave you feeling quite satiated. Many studies have found connections between nuts and successful weight loss, probably because nuts are so satisfying. Eat them with a meal or snack, and you'll fight off hunger for quite a while.

Nut milks, such as almond milk, are made with nuts, and have been growing in popularity lately. I'm a fan of almond milk myself, and use it in my post-workout protein shakes. It's important to understand exactly what is—and isn't—in nut milks. Manufacturers make nut milks by combining ground nuts and water, and then straining out any solids that remain from the nuts. Although you may think nut milk is high in protein, it actually is not, because it contains mostly water with just a trace of nuts. However, some brands do add protein to their nut milks, as well as nutrients such as calcium, vitamin D, and vitamin E, which is good. Unfortunately, they may also add sugar. If you buy nut milk, be sure to choose a brand that is unsweetened and enriched with protein, vitamin D, and calcium, especially if you drink it regularly as a replacement for milk.

Nuts, nut butters, and seeds are an important part of the Mojito Diet. Enjoy walnuts, almonds, pistachios, pecans, macadamia nuts, and peanuts (which are technically legumes, not nuts, but deliver the health benefits of nuts, so that's how we categorize them) as well as the "butters" made by grinding these nuts into a paste. And don't forget about seeds, including sunflower seeds, flaxseeds, chia seeds, pumpkin seeds, sesame seeds, and pomegranate seeds.

Keep this in mind when you eat nuts and seeds: Although they're super-nutritious, they are also high in calories, so you can't eat them to your heart's content. Measure your portion sizes to make sure you're eating the right amount. And avoid added salt, which can raise blood pressure, and sweeteners such as sugar, honey, or molasses, which add calories and low-quality carbohydrates.

You'll see when you read the Mojito Diet meal planning guidelines that I place nuts in their own category, rather than counting them as just another protein. I have a good reason for this. Nuts deliver so many health benefits that I want to single them out and encourage you to eat them often—ideally, every day. But if you really don't like nuts, you can substitute other proteins instead.

DR. JUAN'S WISDOM

GOOD NEWS FOR PLANT-PROTEIN LOVERS

More people are choosing plant-based proteins over meat. Some decide to become vegetarian or vegan; others just want to optimize their health by including more nutrient-rich plant foods in their diet.

If you're looking to swap plant foods for animal foods while following the Mojito Diet, do so with my blessing and my encouragement. The Mojito Diet is flexible and gives you all the space you need to choose whatever kinds of protein you prefer. Just be sure to include protein and fiber in each meal and snack.

Do keep in mind, though, that vegans sometimes find it difficult to get enough iron, calcium, vitamin D, vitamin B_{12}, zinc, and omega-3 fatty acids. Fortunately, supplements can help fill in. Talk with your doctor about whether you need them.

Soy

There have been so many health claims made about soy foods such as tofu, tempeh, soy milk, miso, edamame, and soy-based meat replacement foods. But further research has failed to support many of the near-miraculous promises made about soy foods and weight loss, cancer, heart disease, and brain health. I'm not surprised, because some of those promises were quite extreme. And some people, such as survivors of hormone-sensitive cancers, are advised to avoid soy.

Here's my position on soy foods: If you like them and your doctor hasn't told you to restrict them, it's fine to include them in your diet. But don't go out of your way to eat them if you aren't crazy about them. Even though soy is a good source of protein, some soy foods are highly processed, and you'd be better off eating less-processed meats, poultry, seafood, beans, or other protein-rich foods. (An exception to this is edamame and roasted soy nuts.) Go ahead and have tofu and soy milk if you enjoy them, but don't bother with soy dogs, soy "meats," and other highly processed soy foods. If you choose soy milk over dairy milk, be sure to select a low-fat variety that is fortified with vitamin D and calcium, and that doesn't have added sweeteners or flavorings.

Eat This to Halt Hunger

Both protein and fiber satisfy your appetite, but they're even more effective when paired. The best way to feel satiated for hours is to combine protein and fiber—which is what we do with all of the meals and snacks in the Mojito Diet. Together, protein and fiber satisfy your hunger better and longer than either one can on its own. Some super-filling protein/fiber combinations include:

- Peanut butter on whole grain bread
- An apple and a handful of almonds
- Cheese and whole grain crackers
- Yogurt and blueberries
- Beans and brown rice
- Whole grain cereal with milk
- Peanut butter on a banana
- Carrots dipped in hummus
- Chili with beans
- A hard-boiled egg and blackberries

- Cottage cheese and a peach

- A smoothie made with berries, mango, and yogurt or milk

- A veggie-stuffed omelet

- A salad topped with chicken or seafood

Pass the Guacamole: Fat Is Back on the Menu

For many years, conventional wisdom said that all dietary fat was bad for heart health and weight gain. People were told that eating fat would make them fat, and that cutting out as much fat as possible by eating low-fat diets would help their hearts. Beginning in the 1990s, an avalanche of fat-free products, such as fat-free cookies and cakes, showed up in grocery stores, promising to make us thin and reduce heart disease. Ironically, the opposite occurred, because all those fat-free products replaced fat with refined carbohydrates that actually contributed to the obesity epidemic, rather than reversing it.

We know much more about fat today. For example, we know that fats in seafood, nuts (especially walnuts), seeds, olives and olive oil, avocados, and some other kinds of foods are actually quite good for our hearts. It's really just the saturated fat in animal foods, especially fatty meats, butter, lard, and shortening, that appears to be linked to heart disease and other health problems. I also recommend avoiding or limiting coconut oil and palm and palm kernel oils because they contain saturated fat.

Drastically cutting fat from your diet is harmful because your body needs some fat for optimal health. Heart-healthy fats can help lower the artery-clogging LDL ("bad") cholesterol in your blood, may reduce inflammation, and could reduce type 2 diabetes risk by having a positive effect on blood sugar and insulin.

As you start following the Mojito Diet, you'll find plenty of avocado in the menus and recipes. Avocado is an important ingredient in Latin cuisine, but what gives it an even more beloved place in my heart is that it's an incredibly nutritious food. Avocado contains a long list of nutrients, including fiber, potassium, antioxidants, B vitamins, and vitamins C, E, and K, to name a few. It is also a wonderful source of heart-healthy monounsaturated fat. Cooks love avocado because it's so versatile, and can do so much more than just take the lead role in your favorite guacamole recipe. Avocado can substitute for butter on toast, add flavor to salads, fill up a sandwich or wrap, and provide deliciousness to smoothies and sauces. One of my favorite ways to eat avocado is to chop it up, combine it with mango, red onion, and diced jalapeños, and spoon it onto a beautiful piece of baked salmon.

You don't want to eat too much fat, though—even if it's heart-healthy, fat is high in calories and can contribute to weight gain. By following the Mojito Diet, you'll get the right amount of the healthiest kinds of fat.

DR. JUAN'S WISDOM

HAVE YOUR CHOLESTEROL CHECKED

I recommend having your cholesterol checked at least once a year. When you do, your test results will include several different numbers. Cholesterol is measured in mg/dL, which stands for milligrams per deciliter. Here's what the test results mean:

TOTAL CHOLESTEROL
Desirable: Under 200 mg/dL. *Borderline high:* 200 to 239. *High:* 240 or above.

HDL ("GOOD") CHOLESTEROL
Ideal (most protective against heart disease): 60 or higher. *Moderate:* 40 to 59. *Low (major risk factor for heart disease):* Less than 40.

LDL ("BAD") CHOLESTEROL
Optimal: Less than 100. *Near optimal:* 100 to 129. *Borderline high:* 130 to 159. *High:* 160 to 189. *Very high:* 190 or above.

TRIGLYCERIDES
Normal: Less than 150. *Borderline high:* 150 to 199. *High:* 200 to 499. *Very high:* 500 or above.

MOJITO DIET SUCCESS STORY: MARIA

Losing Weight While Having Diabetes

Maria has struggled with her weight all her life. She was obese as a child and has type 1 diabetes. She has managed to get in control of her weight as an adult, but weight gain is always a concern. "I'm a motivational speaker, I appear often on television, and I host my own show, Maria Marin Live on Facebook," Maria says. "I have to look good and watch my weight."

After putting on some extra pounds over the holidays, Maria, fifty, needed to make some changes. So she gave the Mojito Diet a try. She was surprised by how much she liked it, and how quickly she began to see results. During her first ten days on the Mojito Diet, Maria lost seven pounds; within a few weeks, she met her goal of losing fifteen pounds.

"I especially liked the first week, Grain Drop, so much," Maria says. "When I eat too many grains I immediately start to gain weight, so cutting out grains for a week had a big impact. I lost weight and my blood sugar went down. I even needed less insulin."

Maria had followed low-carbohydrate diets before, but they typically cut out fruit as well as grains. She likes that the Mojito Diet allows several servings of fruit each day, because eating fruit satisfies her sweet tooth.

"In the past, in order to lose weight I cut out all carbs, including fruit. I thought I had to do that. But when Dr. Juan told me it was okay to eat fruit I trusted him and gave it a try," Maria says. "I was thrilled that I could lose weight while having fruit."

Getting enough protein can be a challenge for Maria, who considers herself an "almost vegetarian" who hardly ever eats meat or fish. However, she loves beans, nuts, and eggs, and appreciates that the Mojito Diet makes it easy to build meals around those powerful proteins.

And, like so many people who follow the Mojito Diet, Maria is a huge fan of Mojito Water. "I've told everyone I know about Mojito Water—if you come to my place, I'll serve you Mojito Water," Maria says. "I never used to drink enough water, but now I get all the water I need. I mix up a pitcher, pour a big glass, put it next to my computer, and next thing I know, it's empty."

7

Eat Bread Again! Carbohydrates Can Help with Weight Loss

When I was growing up in Puerto Rico, nearly every meal I ate was packed with carbohydrates. For breakfast, my family and I would typically eat bread such as *mallorca*, a sweet, eggy pastry topped with powdered sugar. I loved *mallorcas*! I don't know a Puerto Rican who doesn't. Lunch might have been empanadas—a deep-fried dough stuffed with meat, spices, onions, and peppers—or deep-fried fritters made with taro root, plantains, and pork. Dinner often featured white rice, which plays a starring role in so many traditional Puerto Rican dishes. A plate of bread, rolls, or cornbread always had a place on my family's dinner table. And to satisfy my father's sweet tooth, my mother served a dessert (or two) every evening.

Of course, we also had the usual high-carbohydrate American foods in our house—pizza, spaghetti, sugary cereal, and all the rest. I can feel my blood sugar going up just thinking about all those carb-laden foods. A high-carb diet wasn't particular to my family or to Puerto Rican cuisine during my childhood—the chances are pretty good that you probably had a carbohydrate-heavy upbringing too.

For a long time, nutrition experts believed that all dietary fat was bad, so they pushed carbohydrates as a replacement for fat. What a mistake. As Americans loaded up on carbohydrates—especially refined grains like white bread, white flour, and white rice—heart disease rates went up rather than down, and Americans' waistlines grew larger. As obesity rates increased, nutritionists suspected that the emphasis on carbohydrates was backfiring, and an inevitable reversal began to occur. Low-fat, high-carb diets did not deliver what they had promised. Around the early 2000s, the carbohydrate pendulum took a full swing in the opposite direction, and very low-carbohydrate diets arrived on the scene. These diets won fans because they offered an innovative way to shed excess pounds. Instead of embracing carbohydrates, they dramatically restricted them, focusing primarily on the high-protein, high-fat foods such as beef, lamb, pork, bacon, and sausage that nutrition experts had been telling us to avoid for so many years. Very low-carbohydrate diets typically limit daily carbohydrate intake to as little as 20 grams of carbohydrates per day, which is about the amount you'd get in a single slice of whole wheat bread or a small apple. Compare this with the approximately 300 grams of carbohydrates in an ordinary American diet today and you'll see that very low-carbohydrate diets really are dramatically different from what most people in the United States are eating.

These low-carb, high-protein diets did produce results: Various studies found that they tended to result in higher short-term weight loss than low-fat, high-carbohydrate diets. For a while, they were held up as the holy grail of weight loss, because they seemed to work better than other kinds of diets. But then, as researchers looked more closely at some of these diets, problems started to appear.

What You Lose with Very Low-Carb Diets

It is true that very low-carbohydrate diets do help people lose weight. But they absolutely are not the long-term solution that we need for permanent weight loss. I have watched with great interest as many of my patients have tried following very low-carb diets, and it hasn't gone well. Here's how it typically goes for them.

At first, they enjoy success, losing some weight and raving about how wonderful it is that they can eat nearly unlimited amounts of meat. Then, after a few weeks—or for some of them, even just a few days—they start to get very tired of all that protein and fat and begin to crave the fruit, milk, bread, and grains that have been banished from their daily meal plans. They also start to experience some of the unpleasant side effects of very low-carbohydrate diets, such as headache, fatigue, constipation, and bad breath. Frustrated, they start to "cheat" on their diet, sneaking some of the bread and fruit and other carb-rich foods they are forbidden to eat. Before they know it, they've given up on the diet and have regained their lost weight.

In my view, the fatal flaw of highly restrictive, very low-carbohydrate diets is that, although they do produce weight loss, they are so hard to follow that people just can't stick with them for the long term. They regain their lost weight and have nothing to show for their efforts. Plus, such diets tend to rely too heavily on meat, including processed and fatty red meats. As we discussed in chapter 6, it's okay to have these kinds of meats occasionally, but it's best to focus on healthier, leaner protein sources.

And then there are the disagreeable side effects that very low-carbohydrate diets can cause. Dramatically cutting carbs can trigger a process in the body known as ketosis. When carbohydrates are in short supply and your body doesn't have glucose to use for energy, it turns instead to stored body fat as fuel. Although this may sound like a good idea—we all want to burn body fat, right?—it can result in annoying ketosis-related side effects such as headache, nausea, fatigue, and bad breath as acid builds up in your blood. There's even something called "keto flu," which is a group of flu-like symptoms caused by ketosis. Some diet experts believe that inducing ketosis on a regular basis is a good way to lose weight, but I don't buy it—I think the risks outweigh the benefits.

To me, very low-carbohydrate diets are too extreme. They cut out important nutrients found in high-quality carbohydrates, typically rely too heavily on meat, and are too difficult to follow on a long-term basis. And science has not shown that they are safer or more successful over time than more reasonable diets. That's why, rather than going to an anti-carb extreme, I recommend a more balanced strategy, one that embraces the positives of a lower-carbohydrate approach while letting go of the negatives.

When I designed the Mojito Diet, I wanted to create an eating plan that offers a balance between the advantages and the challenges of a low-carbohydrate diet—a plan that keeps the high-quality carbohydrates while sidelining the low-quality ones. Although drastically cutting back on carbs isn't the way to go, limiting them in an intelligent way and focusing on better-quality carbohydrates does have advantages and can bring about healthy weight loss.

And so, with the Mojito Diet, I have created what I consider to be a perfect balance of high-quality carbohydrates, protein, and fat. This strategy helps you lose weight, lower your risk of disease, and enjoy your food. It offers you a sensible way to cut back on carbs overall while still leaving room for the better-quality carbohydrates that your body needs.

DR. JUAN'S WISDOM

HAVE YOUR BLOOD SUGAR CHECKED

If you haven't had your blood sugar tested in the past twelve months, I recommend making an appointment with your doctor to have it checked. There are several kinds of laboratory blood tests used to check blood sugar. The most commonly used are the HbA1c test (also known as the A1c test), the fasting plasma glucose, and the oral glucose tolerance test. Blood sugar is measured in milligrams per deciliter (mg/dL). Here's what the results of these three kinds of diabetes blood tests mean:

HBA1C

Normal: Less than 5.7 percent. *Prediabetes:* 5.7 to 6.4 percent. *Diabetes:* 6.5 percent or higher.

FASTING PLASMA GLUCOSE

Normal: Under 100 mg/dL. *Prediabetes:* 100 to 125. *Diabetes:* 126 or higher.

ORAL GLUCOSE TOLERANCE TEST

Normal: Less than 140. *Prediabetes:* 140 to 199. *Diabetes:* 200 or higher.

The Good You Gain from Carbohydrates

I agree that there are carbohydrates we should be cutting back on. I'm talking about you, sugar. And white flour. And all the foods made with sugar and white flour, such as white bread and white pasta, as well as refined grains. And even my beloved *mallorcas*! These foods contain low-quality carbohydrates. It's okay to have them occasionally, as rare indulgences, but generally it's best to limit them.

The truth is, our bodies need high-quality carbohydrates for optimal health, just as they need lean protein and healthy fats. We can't just cut out all carbs and expect to function in a healthy way. When you eat carbohydrates, your body breaks them down and converts them to glucose, or blood sugar, which goes into your blood to be circulated throughout your body. Insulin helps deliver blood sugar to your cells, tissues, and organs; this is the energy your body needs to function well.

Although we typically think of carbohydrates as being found in breads, cereals, pasta, and other grain-based foods, they're also in vegetables, fruit, dairy foods, legumes, seeds, and nuts. We're better off avoiding white bread and other low-quality refined carbohydrates, which have few or no nutrients; but there are many very healthy foods rich in high-quality carbohydrates that have an important place in a nutritious diet. When people follow very low-carb diets that cut out these healthy foods, they may lose weight temporarily, but they trade short-term gain for a long-term loss by putting themselves at risk of developing deficiencies in certain vitamins and minerals. That's why the Mojito Diet includes enough high-quality carbohydrates to give you these very important nutrients.

When you follow the Mojito Diet, you'll be getting balanced amounts of good carbohydrates—and you'll be benefiting from some important nutrients found in these foods, including fiber, antioxidants, vitamins, and minerals. Here's why these nutrients are so important, for both weight loss and overall health.

Fiber: The Carbohydrate Superstar

Dietary fiber is one of several types of carbohydrate found in plant foods, and it's one of the most beneficial. Also referred to as roughage, dietary fiber not only helps you feel full and stay satiated after eating—which is a huge bonus when you're trying to lose weight—but it helps reduce the risk of various diseases and health conditions, including heart disease. There are two types of dietary fiber: soluble and insoluble. Each has important health benefits, and many foods contain both kinds of fiber.

Soluble fiber, which can be dissolved in water, is broken down by bacteria in your intestines. As it travels through your digestive system, it absorbs water and becomes sludgy and gelatin-like—not a pretty thing to envision, but quite advantageous for your intestines. This sludgy gel slows down the rate at which your stomach empties, which is why it helps you feel full after a meal. It also slows the absorption of sugar into your blood, which helps keep blood sugar stable. Slower digestion also gives your body more time to absorb the nutrients in the foods you've eaten. Not bad for a mess of gloppy sludge.

DR. JUAN'S WISDOM

WHAT ARE GRAINS?

What am I talking about when I refer to "grains" in the Mojito Diet? I use the term to cover any foods made with wheat, rice, oats, quinoa, barley, and cornmeal, as well as other less common types of grains. Examples include bread, rice, oatmeal, pasta, tortillas, breakfast cereals, bagels, muffins, cake, crackers, and so on. During the first week of the Mojito Diet, you'll follow the Grain Drop plan, during which you won't eat any grains at all. But you'll add grains back into your daily meal plan when you follow the Clean 16 Fast during Week 2. I encourage you to choose whole grains whenever possible, such as whole grain bread, whole grain cereal, brown rice, and whole grain crackers.

Another benefit of soluble fiber—one that warms my cardiologist heart—is that it binds with fatty acids, which helps block the absorption of LDL ("bad") cholesterol in your body. Picture it so: Soluble fiber acts kind of like a vacuum that pulls cholesterol out of your body and gets rid of it in your stool. Eat foods with soluble fiber on a regular basis and you could see your LDL go down, which is exactly what we want for improving heart health.

Some great sources of soluble fiber include whole grains (especially oat bran and oatmeal), vegetables (especially brussels sprouts, broccoli, and cabbage), nuts, beans, dried peas, lentils, fruits (especially apples, pears, and citrus fruit), and seeds.

The other kind of dietary fiber is insoluble fiber. As its name suggests, it doesn't dissolve in water, so it passes through your intestines pretty much without being digested. Think apple peels, sesame seed hulls, and the fibrous stems of spinach and kale. Having those foods go through you without breaking down is a good thing because it bulks your stool and helps prevent constipation by keeping your bowel movements regular.

Insoluble fiber is found in fruits (especially those with edible peels, such as apples and pears, or edible seeds, such as raspberries), vegetables, nuts, seeds, and whole grains (especially wheat bran).

Fiber-rich diets have been linked to improved cholesterol levels, a reduced risk of heart disease and stroke, and lower blood pressure. Eating fiber can have a huge impact on your blood sugar—in fact, studies have found that eating a low-fiber diet can double the risk of type 2 diabetes. In addition to slowing the absorption of sugar into the blood, eating fiber-rich foods can prevent blood sugar spikes that lead to hunger and carbohydrate cravings soon after eating. It may also lower your chance of developing certain gastrointestinal conditions such as colorectal cancer and, perhaps, other types of cancer.

Unfortunately, most of us don't get enough fiber—and if you follow a very low-carbohydrate diet, you're unlikely to get the dietary fiber you need. Americans eat an average of only 16 grams of fiber daily, but the recommended daily intake of fiber is:

- Men age fifty and under: 38 grams
- Men over age fifty: 30 grams
- Women age fifty and under: 25 grams
- Women over age fifty: 21 grams

DR. JUAN'S WISDOM

EAT THIS FOR FIBER

The following foods are among the best sources of dietary fiber:

- High-fiber bran cereal
- Beans (especially navy beans, white beans, yellow beans, cranberry beans, adzuki beans, garbanzo beans, pinto beans, black beans, lima beans, great northern beans, kidney beans, and soybeans)
- Peas (especially split peas, pigeon peas, cowpeas/black-eyed peas, and green peas)
- Shredded wheat–type breakfast cereal
- Wheat bran flake–type breakfast cereal
- Lentils
- Artichokes
- Pears and apples
- Seeds (especially pumpkin seeds and chia seeds)
- Avocados
- Bulgur
- Berries (especially raspberries and blackberries)
- Collard greens
- Sweet potatoes baked with their skin
- White potatoes baked with their skin
- Popcorn
- Almonds
- Whole wheat spaghetti

A Fantastic Fuel for Weight Loss

Here's the cool thing about fiber: if you haven't been getting enough, you can start to change that right away. Following the Mojito Diet is very likely to boost your fiber intake into a much healthier range because it includes plenty of fruit, vegetables, legumes, nuts, and seeds, and a reasonable amount of whole grains.

Many studies have found a link between fiber and weight loss. One of my favorites was published in the *Annals of Internal Medicine* in 2015. In the study, researchers asked 240 overweight adults with metabolic syndrome to follow high-fiber diets. The researchers wanted to see if eating more fiber would help study participants lose weight and keep it off.

Half of the study volunteers received a full eating plan that recommended thirteen different dietary changes, one of which was to eat more fiber. Not surprisingly, that group lost weight. But here's the really interesting part of the study's findings: The other half of the study participants were simply told to try to eat 30 grams of fiber a day. That's it. They didn't receive a whole big eating plan or diet protocol with a dozen recommendations. They weren't even told to cut back on calories. All they received was one single piece of advice: to try to eat 30 grams of fiber a day.

The results were pretty amazing. The study participants who did nothing more than eat more fiber lost an average of about five pounds, and they kept it off for the full length of the study, which was twelve months. They achieved these results even without hitting their fiber targets every day. Although they were told to aim for 30 grams of fiber daily, they took in an average of only 19 grams a day, or about what you'd get in two slices of whole wheat bread (6 grams), an apple (4 grams), a half cup of black beans (6 grams), and an ounce of almonds (3 grams). Think about that: These people basically lost weight without really trying or knowingly cutting back on how much they ate. But because they increased their fiber intake, they felt less hungry and ate less food without even realizing it. And here's a bonus: In addition to losing weight, the study participants lowered their blood pressure and improved their insulin response.

Imagine what you can do if you eat more fiber *and* try to place some limits on how much you eat! Weight loss truly is within your reach.

The bottom line? Cutting out all carbohydrates isn't the answer. Instead, eating high-fiber, high-quality carbohydrate foods is a crucial part of a successful weight-loss strategy—which is why we embrace it in the Mojito Diet and include many delicious high-fiber foods in your daily eating plan. As you follow the Mojito Diet, be sure to eat all of the fruits, vegetables, nuts, legumes, seeds, and whole grains recommended in each day's menus. Doing so truly will help you reach your weight-loss goals.

From A to Zinc and Beyond

Eating a very low-carbohydrate diet can prevent you from getting enough of the vitamins and minerals you need, because some of these important nutrients are found primarily in good-quality carbohydrate-rich foods such as the fruits, vegetables, whole grains, dairy, legumes, nuts, and seeds that very low-carb diets limit or eliminate. But when you eat a wide range of vitamin- and mineral-rich carbohydrate-containing foods, as you will with the Mojito Diet, you'll make your body happy by giving it plenty of the nutrients that are crucial for good health.

In addition to vitamins and minerals, carbohydrate-rich foods can deliver substances known as antioxidants. Here's what they can do for you:

The cells in your body are subjected to all kinds of normal damage on an everyday basis. Some of that damage comes from free radicals, which are by-products created when the body uses oxygen, or when you are exposed to environmental toxins such as air pollution, excessive sunlight, or cigarette smoke. Free radicals can cause damage known as oxidative stress, which can harm cells throughout your body. Over time, this oxidative stress is believed to contribute to cancer, heart disease, stroke, Alzheimer's disease, diabetes, Parkinson's disease, age-related macular degeneration, and other conditions.

Lucky for us, antioxidants can shield our cells from some of the oxidative stress that bombards them each day. Like firefighters called in to douse flames, antioxidants can protect cells by delaying or stopping disease-producing cell damage from occurring.

Antioxidants are found in many fruits and vegetables, as well as some nonplant foods such as eggs and salmon. (They are also found in vitamin supplements, but antioxidants generally appear to work much more effectively in food rather than pills.) Some powerhouse antioxidants include vitamin A, vitamin C, vitamin E, anthocyanins, beta-carotene, catechins, lipoic acid, lutein, lycopene, selenium, and zeaxanthin.

Don't worry, you don't have to know all about the various antioxidants and where to find them. The easiest way to get the optimal protection from a wide range of antioxidants—both the ones we know about and the ones that may yet be discovered—is to eat a wide range of plant foods, as you will when following the Mojito Diet.

Let your eyes guide you as you shop for produce, because different-colored fruits and vegetables tend to have different types of antioxidants—for example, yellow and orange produce such as corn, carrots, yellow and orange peppers, and cantaloupe are excellent sources of the antioxidants zeaxanthin and lutein, which have been linked to eye health, whereas dark-green vegetables such as kale and spinach serve up antioxidant vitamins A, C, and E. The best way to get all the antioxidants you need is to eat a rainbow of plant foods, especially these red, purple, green, yellow, and orange choices:

- Berries: Blackberries, blueberries, cranberries, elderberries, goji berries, raspberries, strawberries

- Other fruit: Apples (with skin), bananas, cherries, citrus fruits, guava, mango, nectarines, peaches, plums, red grapes

- Vegetables: Artichokes, asparagus, beets, broccoli, brussels sprouts, corn, kale, peppers, spinach, sweet potatoes, tomatoes

- Nuts: Almonds, hazelnuts, pecans, pistachios, walnuts

- Seeds: Flaxseed, sesame, sunflower

- Legumes: Black beans, kidney beans, lentils, pinto beans, red beans, soybeans

- Herbs and spices: Basil, cilantro, cinnamon, clove, cumin, ginger, mint, oregano, parsley, thyme, turmeric

- Chocolate: Cocoa powder, dark chocolate

DR. JUAN'S WISDOM

MINT UP WITH THE MOJITO'S SUPERSTAR INGREDIENT

When you drink a mojito made with mint, you're not just enjoying a refreshing treat—you're also getting a dose of one of the most powerful antioxidants. Mint contains blockbuster levels of antioxidants, according to a scientific analysis of the oxygen radical absorbance capacity (ORAC) score of hundreds of different foods. Of all the foods tested, mint has one of the highest ORAC scores recorded. Other herbs and spices also weigh in with very high ORAC scores.

Don't just wait for your mojito days to enjoy the flavor and antioxidant power of mint and other herbs. Add herbs and spices to all kinds of foods, from breakfast smoothies to lunchtime soups and salads, from salsas to dinner dishes. Start with the recommendations in my Mojito Diet recipes, and go from there.

Herbs and spices are a delicious way to add health-boosting antioxidants to almost any food or recipe. You can buy fresh herbs at most grocery stores. Or else pick up some plants at your local nursery, set them on a sunny windowsill, and enjoy fresh-cut herbs anytime you need them.

Carbohydrates in the Mojito Diet

I hope that by now I have convinced you that following a very low-carbohydrate diet is not the way to go, either for long-term weight loss or for overall health. Instead, I hope you see the benefits of a balanced approach that includes healthy amounts of high-quality carbohydrates and reduces your reliance on the low-quality carbs that may be making up a big part of your diet right now.

I'll tell you all the specific details about each of the Mojito Diet's plans in part 3, but in general, here's how we handle carbohydrates in the Mojito Diet.

During Week 1, you'll follow my Grain Drop plan. For seven days, in addition to protein and fat, you will eat fruits, vegetables, legumes, nuts, and seeds—which provide lots of high-quality carbohydrates—but you *won't* eat any grain-based foods. You'll cut out grains during Week 1 for two reasons: First, doing so will help jump-start your weight loss; and second, it will help you break your dependence on refined white grains and open you up to the delicious taste of whole grains.

During Week 2 of the Mojito Diet, you'll add grains back into your daily menus, but I'll ask you to choose whole grains (such as whole wheat bread, brown rice, and whole grain pasta) rather than refined white grains. Taking a week off from all grains, as you do in the Week 1 Grain Drop plan, prepares you to make the switch to whole grains and to enjoy and appreciate their delicious taste. Making this swap after a week without any grains is easier, because you are so happy to be eating grains again that you are unlikely to mind the difference in taste!

If you're accustomed to eating refined grains such as white bread and white rice, whole grains may take a little getting used to. Whole grains and foods made with them tend to be a little chewier and nuttier than refined grains; if you've only eaten white bread, whole wheat bread will taste a bit different to you. However, I'm confident that you'll soon come to love the toasty flavor of whole grains much more than the bland taste of their white counterparts. After making the switch to whole grain bread, for example, many of my patients tell me they could never go back to the blandness of white bread.

Here's how refined white grains are different from whole grains. Whole grains consist of a grain seed, or kernel, which is made up of three main parts: the bran (the grain's outer layer), the endosperm (the middle layer), and the germ (the inner layer). Whole grains—particularly the bran and germ—are a rich source of fiber, vitamins, and minerals. During the refining process, germ and bran are removed. Although most whole grains tend to be a toasty tan color, refined grains are typically white because so much of their natural goodness has been removed. (To make up for this, white grain products often have vitamins and minerals added back in through a process known as enrichment—but make no mistake, these added nutrients leave much to be desired.) Examples of refined grains and grain products include white rice and white flour, as well as breads, tortillas, cereals, crackers, and pastas made with refined white flour. Most cookies, cakes, and pies are made with refined flours.

By following the Mojito Diet's very sensible approach to carbohydrates, you'll receive all of the many benefits of whole grains while still enjoying the weight-loss advantages that come from including protein at every meal and snack and limiting your overall carb intake. And you'll be taking some very big steps toward optimizing your health. I call that a win-win carbohydrate strategy that everyone can love!

Try These Whole Grains

You may be familiar with a few better-known whole grains, such as whole wheat, brown rice, and oats. But there are many others to enjoy. Consider experimenting with these super-healthy whole grains: amaranth, barley, buckwheat, bulgur, millet, quinoa, triticale, and wild rice. You'll find that some of the recipes in this book include grains you may not have tried before. Now's your chance to see how delicious they are.

You can steam whole grains as you do with rice—check the package for directions, as some take longer than others. Once they're cooked, toss them in a bowl and festoon them with all kinds of other ingredients—beans, vegetables, meat, seafood, salsa, fresh herbs, avocado, shredded cheese, even fresh fruit, such as mango. Making a "grain bowl" for lunch or dinner is an easy way to have a delicious high-fiber meal—and to use up the leftovers in your refrigerator.

To save time, cook a big pot of quinoa, barley, or another grain on the weekend; then divide it into single servings and freeze it to use during the week. Heat it up in the microwave and it's good to go in just minutes, either as a side dish or as the foundation for a grain bowl.

Be sure to look for whole grains as ingredients in bread and other grain-based foods. Just make sure the word *whole* appears in the ingredient list with the grain, to guarantee you're getting all of the grain's nutritional benefit. Some bread manufacturers try to trick consumers by selling "wheat bread" that doesn't actually contain any whole wheat, although it does have a brownish coloring added to make it *look* like whole wheat bread. Don't be fooled. Always check the food label to make sure the grains in the product are whole.

DR. JUAN'S WISDOM

THINK TWICE BEFORE DROPPING GLUTEN

Gluten, a protein in wheat, rye, barley, and triticale, has gotten a lot of attention lately. It's blamed for all kinds of health problems, from digestive complaints and brain fog to miscarriage, depression, and headache. Yikes! If it's that bad, should you stop eating it?

Probably not. I'm not at all convinced that gluten is a nutritional bad guy that everyone should avoid. In fact, unless you have celiac disease or a true intolerance to gluten, I see no reason to leave it out of your diet.

Going gluten-free can be inconvenient and expensive, and when you replace gluten-containing breads and cereals with gluten-free versions, you're likely to get a lot less fiber and a lot more sugar and fat. You'll also be eating much more white rice, which is ground up and used to replace wheat flour in many gluten-free foods. Stop eating gluten if it makes you sick—but if it doesn't, I see no reason to avoid it.

MOJITO DIET SUCCESS STORY: **MARI**

Getting Back in Shape After Having Children

Gaining weight had never been a problem for Mari, a thirty-four-year-old stay-at-home mom and former lab technician. Growing up she had always enjoyed sports and considered herself "skinny." But after having two children in under two years and being so busy with motherhood that she stopped exercising for four years, Mari saw her body changing. "I wasn't happy with the way I looked and felt," she says.

Mari wanted to improve her eating habits and feel like herself again. "I wanted to be able to fit in smaller clothes and also have more energy to play with my kids and go to the gym," she says. She had tried a couple of other diets, including a plan that required users to buy packaged foods, but she hated the way the food tasted. So she decided to give the Mojito Diet a try.

After four months on the Mojito Diet, Mari is thrilled to report that she has lost twelve pounds, burned off 8 percent of her body fat, reduced her waist size by five inches, and come down two dress sizes.

One of her favorite things about the Mojito Diet is that it's easy to follow. "It gives you recipes that are simple to make at home, and it's easy to follow the plan when you eat out," Mari says. "I love that you can eat cheese and also that you can eat half of a small potato; it's very easy to manage the proteins, and I love the Mojito Water!" She enjoys looking forward to reward mojitos at the end of the week, and likes the fact that the Mojito Diet is a fourteen-day plan that can be repeated as many times as needed until your goal weight is reached.

"The Mojito Diet has changed the way I eat and cook," Mari says. "It has made me conscious of my health, and now I'm very aware of what I eat. I feel more energetic and feel like my old self again. After having my two kids I wasn't feeling that good with the way I looked, but now I look and feel much better."

8

~~~~~

Use Sixteen-Hour Fasting to Lose Weight and Improve Health

One of my patients, a fifty-four-year-old lawyer named Margaret, had a heck of a time losing weight. She had been putting on weight since she went through menopause—not a lot, but a few pounds here and a few pounds there. Despite trying several different diets and adding in more exercise, she just couldn't manage to shed the fifteen pounds that had crept up on her during the previous few years. But then she tried something completely different: fasting. Three days a week, she would fast for sixteen hours at a stretch. She ate nothing from 8 p.m. at night until lunchtime the next day. Fasting turned out to be Margaret's weight-loss silver bullet, the strategy that made her excess pounds start to drop off. A couple of months after she started fasting, Margaret got to her goal weight, and she continues to maintain her weight loss by fasting a day or two each week.

When I created the Mojito Diet, I wanted it to include fasting because I know it works. Not only does it help with weight loss, but it may bring about other health benefits as well. The more I learned about the health and weight-loss benefits of fasting, the more I realized it had to be part of my plan.

When you think of fasting, you probably imagine going all day without eating. That's certainly one way to fast, but much of the research being done on fasting for weight loss is discovering that we can benefit from fasting without starving ourselves for a whole day at a time. Instead of not eating for long periods, intermittent fasting—or functional fasting, as I refer to it—alternates occasional periods of fasting with periods of eating. Fasting periods can be as short as sixteen hours, and they typically include the eight hours spent sleeping, which makes the fasting time seem shorter. During my Clean 16 Fast, you will do three nonconsecutive days of sixteen-hour fasts. These fasts are easier than they sound, starting after dinner (by 8 p.m.) and ending at lunchtime the next day.

After considering the pros and cons of various kinds of fasting strategies, I created the Clean 16 Fast because it offers the best combination of practicality and results. It's easy to follow, and it can have a positive impact on weight loss, belly fat, inflammation, insulin resistance, and brain health.

Fasting is a relatively simple way to eat less and increase your weight loss. When you do a sixteen-hour fast—as I recommend with the Clean 16 Fast during Week 2 of the Mojito Diet—you automatically reduce the number of calories you take in, as long as you don't eat more later in the day to make up for the skipped meal.

What's nice about sixteen-hour fasting is that once you get accustomed to doing it three times a week, it begins to feel natural, and it's a relatively easy way to eat less. Some of my patients report feeling intellectually sharper on mornings that they are skipping breakfast, and some have found that they prefer working out on an empty stomach because they feel better physically without a belly full of food.

How Does Fasting Help?

The simplest explanation for why fasting works is that it helps you eat less and take in fewer calories, especially if you don't overeat during nonfasting periods. This can lead to a reduction in weight—and, once you do lose weight, help you keep it off.

Fasting also may help lower the risk of certain diseases. One recent study found that fasting lowered blood pressure, inflammation, blood sugar, triglycerides, and overall blood cholesterol, as well as a hormone that is associated with aging-related changes. In addition, fasting may help your body use blood sugar more effectively by improving the ability of insulin to deliver blood sugar to cells.

Fasting also helps with fat burning. When you fast, you don't provide your body with new fuel, so it has to rely on stored fuel — in other words, the fat that is socked away in your belly, butt, and other jiggly places.

When you fast, you take a break from eating. Why would that be good for your health? One theory is that fasting causes mild stress in your cells, and that stress may strengthen your cells' ability to resist disease. Think of it as the old saying "what doesn't kill you makes you stronger" being applied to cells, rather than people. Occasional fasting also appears to reduce inflammation throughout the body and slow down oxidation, a process that contributes to the aging of cells.

Studies have found links between fasting and a reduction in heart disease risk. Whether this connection is due to weight loss or a cooling down of inflammation or a reduction of oxidation is hard to determine, but I believe the science is strong enough in favor of fasting that I feel comfortable recommending it.

Some studies also suggest that fasting could help delay the onset of Alzheimer's symptoms. The research on this is still in its infancy, and most of it has been done on animals, but there is reason to believe that fasting and calorie restriction could help extend life span, preserve memory, and increase resistance to other age-related diseases. We don't know for sure if fasting would help prevent dementia, or what type of fasting would have the most impact, or which other factors could play a part in dementia prevention.

For example, some studies link fasting with a very low intake of calories overall. Despite all the uncertainty, obesity and insulin resistance do appear to have links to dementia, and it seems likely that losing weight could help the brain. We do know that cardiovascular disease–related defects in the blood vessels of the brain can increase the chances of dementia. I don't think that reducing Alzheimer's risk is, in and of itself, a reason to start fasting. But as someone who has dementia in his family history, I think it's important for researchers to keep looking at whether fasting could help lower its risk.

You may be thinking: "If some fasting is good, wouldn't more fasting be better?" My answer to that is, probably not. If you fast too often or for too long a time, or if you combine fasting with a poor diet on nonfasting days, your efforts could backfire. Too much fasting can slow down your metabolism, pushing your body to hold on to fat rather than to burn it, and interfering with your body's ability to lose weight.

I disagree with fasting plans that alternate long periods of fasting with an unhealthy diet. For example, some fad diets recommend that you eat little or nothing several days a week, and basically eat whatever you want on the other days. Although it's possible this strategy could lead to short-term weight loss, it does nothing to address the quality of your diet. If you're taking in whatever you want on your eating days—cheeseburgers, french fries, sugary soft drinks, and so on—you're not getting the healthy foods that can help improve your health and lower your risk of heart disease, type 2 diabetes, cancer, and other conditions. That's why, on the Mojito Diet, I recommend alternating sixteen-hour fasts with reasonable-size portions of healthy foods.

Fasting isn't for everyone

Some people should avoid fasting for health reasons, or should do so only with their doctor's approval. Fasting isn't recommended if you:

- Are pregnant or breastfeeding

- Take insulin or diabetes medication

- Have a history of disordered eating

- Have liver or kidney disease

- Have hypoglycemia or get weak when you go without eating

If you have type 2 diabetes, check with your doctor before fasting. Personally, I am usually fine with my diabetic patients doing sixteen-hour fasts a couple times a week if they are not on insulin or diabetes medication, because it can be an effective way for them to help lower their overall blood sugar. But you should get your doctor's okay first.

But Isn't Breakfast the Most Important Meal of the Day?

If you're like me, you probably grew up believing that you couldn't skip breakfast because it's the most important meal of the day. You may even have heard of studies showing that people who eat breakfast are less likely to be overweight or obese than those who skip it. So are these things true?

Let's start with what your mother may have told you when she refused to let you leave for school without eating. I agree with her: Children should eat breakfast because it gives them the energy their growing bodies need to learn and process information. Fasting doesn't make sense for kids, whose brains and bodies need fuel on a regular basis. High-sugar breakfasts don't make sense for kids, either—the best combination of foods for children at every meal and snack is protein plus high-fiber carbohydrates and healthy fats.

As for the studies that suggest an association between skipping breakfast and gaining weight, rest assured that there are also studies that show the opposite. Why the mix in findings? It may be that people who tend to eat breakfast also have other healthy habits, such as exercising and choosing nutritious foods. As far as I'm concerned, if you skip breakfast as part of a carefully thought out fasting program like my Clean 16 Fast, you're positioning yourself for successful weight loss. But, on the other hand, if you find that skipping that first meal of the day leaves you so ravenous that you overeat later in the day, fasting might not be the right choice for you. We each have to make the decisions that are best for own bodies. Give it a try, and you may find that it brings weight-loss success that has eluded you in the past, as it did with my patient Margaret.

Tips for Fighting Hunger While Fasting

Some people report feeling hungry when they first start fasting. Once you get into the habit of doing a couple Clean 16 Fasts each week, you'll probably get used to it and won't feel particularly hungry. However, if you do, here are some ways to deal with hunger:

▪ *Fill up with liquid.* While you're fasting, you can drink water, or plain coffee, black tea, or green tea (with no sweetener or milk). You can also make a big pitcher of my Mojito Water (page 198) and drink it in the evening and morning to help fill you up and flush toxins from your body.

▪ *Distract yourself.* Take your mind off hunger pangs by doing some work, reading a book, listening to music, calling a friend, or doing whatever else might absorb your focus and distract you from your hunger.

▪ *Exercise.* Do a ten-minute burst of salsa dancing, go for a walk, play some basketball, or do any other physical activity you enjoy.

▪ *Lean in to the hunger.* This is the opposite of distraction. Instead of trying to take your mind off your hunger, focus on it and become mindful of how it feels and what it represents—not a punishment or a deprivation, but a gift you're giving to your body. Sometimes facing hunger head-on helps you realize that you can handle it, and that you can allow yourself to be hungry without always reaching for food to fill the empty feeling in your stomach and your mind.

▪ *Make sure it's hunger that you're feeling.* That "hungry" feeling you're experiencing may actually be something else—boredom, loneliness, or frustration, for example. Try to study your hunger to determine whether it's physical or emotional. If you discover that emotions rather than an empty stomach are triggering a desire to eat, think about ways that you can satisfy your emotional cravings without turning to food.

▪ *Reframe it.* Imagine ways that you can reframe the feeling of hunger—instead of thinking that it's an emptiness that you don't like, tell yourself that it's the feeling of your body burning up extra fat and calories.

DR. JUAN'S WISDOM

LOOK DEEPER IF HUNGER TRIGGERS ANXIETY

Some people get upset when they feel hunger pangs, and they gobble up food right away rather than allowing themselves to get hungry. They don't just feel uncomfortable when they get hungry—they feel fearful, anxious, and distressed.

If your physical hunger provokes a deep emotional response, try to explore your feelings to understand the thoughts and emotions behind them. Remind yourself that if you're healthy, there's no harm in being hungry for a few hours—it may be slightly unpleasant, but it won't hurt you. However, if your feelings about hunger are complex, cause serious anxiety, or are associated with disordered eating, you might want to consider discussing them with a mental health professional.

MOJITO DIET SUCCESS STORY: DANNY

Transitioning to a Healthier Lifestyle

When Danny started following the Mojito Diet, his goal was not only to lose weight, but to improve the quality of his diet. He had been looking for a way to incorporate more nutritious foods into his meals.

Unfortunately, eating healthy isn't easy for Danny. As a transit armed protective officer, Danny's work schedule makes it challenging for him to eat well. This is a common problem for people who work shifts or irregular schedules. It's easy for them to overeat or to fill up on junk food, and difficult to fit meal-planning and exercise into their erratic hours.

Danny, forty-nine, also wanted to improve his health, and he knew the importance of eating more vegetables. But in the past, finding ways to add more veggies to his diet was a challenge. And so, when he began following the Mojito Diet, he took it as an opportunity to commit to a new way of eating.

Danny has succeeded with both of his goals. Not only has he lost fourteen pounds and trimmed three inches from his waist, but he has significantly improved the quality of his diet. "I do a much better job now of eating healthier meals and having more greens throughout the day," Danny says.

Although Danny wanted to lose weight, he absolutely did not want to have to eat boring foods. For that reason, he appreciates the flavorful recipes that are built into every day of the Mojito Diet meal plan. "I loved the recipes, especially the Brazilian *feijoada*—wow!" Danny says.

9

Eat for Your Heart and Your Mind

I'm always thrilled to see patients who have lost weight. They come into my office for their checkups with huge smiles on their faces and a spring in their step, so excited to tell me about their success. Rather than groaning when they're asked to step onto the scale, they jump on happily, thrilled with their accomplishment. Seeing this is one of the best parts of my job.

As happy as I am to observe my patients' trim, slim physiques, how they look isn't that important to me. As I've said before, I believe people of all sizes and shapes can be attractive, so if it were only about appearance, I wouldn't really care about weight loss. What excites me, as a cardiologist, is the medical test results that these patients typically receive. When they lose weight, they're likely to have lower blood pressure, better cholesterol counts, and lower blood sugar numbers than they had before they lost weight, especially if they followed an eating plan like the Mojito Diet that emphasizes heart-healthy foods and exercise. Those improved test results give me the greatest satisfaction of all!

In my overweight and obese patients, I am especially concerned about high blood pressure, also known as hypertension. As blood travels through the arteries it exerts pressure on them; if the pressure is too high on a regular basis, a diagnosis of hypertension must be made. High blood pressure worries me because it is a contributing cause of death for about 410,000 Americans per year, and is linked to heart disease and stroke, the two leading causes of death in the United States.

High blood pressure can damage your arteries, eventually causing them to bulge, leak, or become blocked. Artery damage triggered by high blood pressure can lead to serious complications, such as aneurysm, heart attack, heart failure, an enlarged heart, stroke, kidney failure, or dementia. It can also cause vision loss, sexual dysfunction, or peripheral artery disease. Believe me, it's better when blood pressure is in a lower, healthier range.

About half of all adults have high blood pressure; in those who are overweight or obese, high blood pressure is even more common, especially as people get older. If you're over fifty and obese, your likelihood of having high blood pressure is about 71 percent; if you're over sixty-five, that probability goes up to about 86 percent.

I kept high blood pressure very much in mind when I designed the Mojito Diet. I wanted to create a diet that would not only help with weight loss, but would assist in lowering high blood pressure too. That's why I based the Mojito Diet in part on the highly respected blood pressure–lowering DASH eating plan.

Although DASH was developed for people with hypertension—it actually stands for Dietary Approaches to Stop Hypertension—it does way more than just lower blood pressure. Many studies have linked the DASH eating plan to weight loss as well as lower blood pressure. For example, the ENCORE study found weight loss of up to nineteen pounds in four months, and blood pressure reductions of up to 16 mmHg (systolic) and 10 mmHg (diastolic) in people following the DASH plan. Study participants who exercised lowered their blood pressure even more than those who didn't. DASH has also been found to lower the risk of gout, type 2 diabetes, and premature death from various causes.

In some studies, people following DASH saw their blood pressure begin to drop within just two weeks of starting their new eating plan. Two weeks! Some blood pressure–lowering medications don't work that quickly!

Picking Up Where DASH Leaves Off

"So, Dr. Juan," you may be thinking, "if you like the DASH eating plan so much, why shouldn't I just follow that instead of the Mojito Diet?" That's a good question! Here's my answer: Since DASH was designed more than twenty years ago, we've learned some very important new lessons about weight loss, blood pressure, fasting, and heart health that are not necessarily reflected in the DASH guidelines.

For example, since that first DASH eating plan was designed, we now have a better understanding of the following:

- The crucial role that protein plays in weight loss

- The importance of focusing on high-quality carbohydrates and cutting back on low-quality carbohydrates for weight loss and heart health

- The contributions that heart-healthy fats can make to a healthy diet

- The fact that that dietary cholesterol in foods such as eggs does not seem to raise blood cholesterol levels or heart disease risk as we once thought it did

- The health and weight-loss benefits of nuts

- The many advantages that plant proteins such as nuts, seeds, beans, peas, and lentils bring to weight loss and overall health, especially when used in place of red meat and processed meat

All of that new knowledge informed my thinking as I decided how to calibrate the Mojito Diet for optimal success. I have incorporated some of DASH's most effective blood pressure–lowering principles into the Mojito Diet, along with new information about weight loss and health. The Mojito Diet starts where DASH leaves off, using the latest nutritional science to create an eating plan that delivers weight loss as well as heart health.

The Mojito Diet and Your Mind

I know I talk a lot about how the Mojito Diet can benefit your heart. What can I say? I'm a cardiologist, and I think about hearts all the time! But I also had your brain in mind when I designed the Mojito Diet, which incorporates many of the foods featured in the MIND diet. The MIND diet was designed to optimize brain health and reduce the risk of Alzheimer's disease.

The MIND diet (MIND stands for the intimidating-sounding Mediterranean-DASH Intervention for Neurodegenerative Delay) is exciting because researchers discovered that it lowered the risk of Alzheimer's disease by as much as 53 percent in people who followed it very closely, and by 35 percent among participants who followed it moderately well. This is excellent news for people like me who have dementia running in their families. Like the MIND plan, the Mojito Diet includes lots of vegetables, fruits, whole grains, and lean protein, while limiting red meat, processed meat, and saturated fat.

If you're eager to take steps to lower your risk of Alzheimer's—as I am—try to include plenty of leafy greens (at least six servings per week of spinach, kale, Swiss chard, romaine, or other greens) and berries (at least two servings per week) in your daily food choices. It's easy to do this in the Mojito Diet, because you can always swap in one vegetable for another or one fruit for another. Unlike the Mojito Diet, the MIND plan includes a glass of wine daily. It also limits cheese to just one serving per week. However, I'm not convinced that limiting cheese so drastically or drinking wine every day is necessary.

I do suggest you keep this in mind, however: Of all the brain-healthy foods included in the MIND diet, blueberries are considered the most potent brain-protecting food of all. This is just one of the reasons I eat blueberries for breakfast almost every morning, and why I include them in the Mojito Diet meal plan often. I love tiny wild blueberries, which are available frozen. Other berries are packed with nutrients too.

As you can see, the Mojito Diet integrates so many best practices from a variety of science-based sources. It's exciting for me to think about all the people whose health and well-being will improve thanks to the Mojito Diet!

HAVE YOUR BLOOD PRESSURE CHECKED

If you haven't had your blood pressure measured in the past twelve months, please make an appointment with your doctor for a checkup. When your blood pressure is measured, ask your doctor or nurse to write it down for you so you know what it is.

Blood pressure is described with two numbers: The top number (systolic) measures pressure when the heart is beating. The bottom number (diastolic) measures pressure when the heart is at rest between beats. Blood pressure is measured in units known as millimeters of mercury, or mmHg. Here's what the numbers mean:

BLOOD PRESSURE CATEGORY	SYSTOLIC (UPPER NUMBER)		DIASTOLIC (LOWER NUMBER)
Normal	Less than 120	and	Less than 80
Elevated	120 to 129	and	Less than 80
High blood pressure, stage 1	130 to 139	or	80 to 89
High blood pressure, stage 2	140 or higher	or	90 or higher
Hypertensive crisis (requires immediate medical attention)	Higher than 180	and/or	Higher than 120

Four Crucial Minerals for Heart Health

Like the DASH plan, the Mojito Diet makes sure you get optimal amounts of four major nutritional minerals that have been linked to blood pressure regulation and heart health: sodium, potassium, magnesium, and calcium. Each is linked, positively or negatively, to high blood pressure risk.

Sodium

When it comes to high blood pressure, a lot of attention goes to sodium, which is the primary ingredient in table salt. Consuming more sodium than your body needs can cause your body to retain water, which can in turn make blood volume and blood pressure go up. Excess sodium can also cause artery walls to become less flexible. Eating less sodium can help lower blood pressure and reduce damage to blood vessels, which is why I limit sodium in the Mojito Diet.

Not everybody has high blood pressure, but it makes good sense for everyone to limit the sodium in their diet and to cut back if they consume it in large amounts. Even if you don't have high blood pressure now, you may eventually develop it. As we age, it's normal for the walls of our blood vessels to become more rigid and less able to handle increases in blood pressure, so even if you do everything "right," your blood pressure may become elevated as the years go by. Therefore I encourage all of my patients—not just those with high blood pressure—to limit sodium. I agree with the American Heart Association's recommendation on sodium: Every American should aim to consume no more than 2,300 milligrams of sodium per day, with an ideal limit of 1,500 milligrams per day, especially if you have high blood pressure.

Here are some simple ways to cut back on sodium:

▪ *Avoid hidden sodium.* You know there's lots of salt in potato chips, tortilla chips, and pretzels, but you probably don't realize that sodium is a hidden ingredient in many foods that we don't think of as being especially salty, such as spaghetti sauce, breakfast cereal, salad dressing, bread, pizza, soup, and cold cuts. Even the rotisserie chickens at your grocery store may contain a surprisingly high amount of sodium. Don't assume that because something doesn't taste very salty, it's low in sodium.

▪ *Choose fresh or plain frozen vegetables.* If you use canned veggies, choose varieties without added salt.

- *Go with whole foods as often as possible.* There's no reason to worry about sodium if you're eating foods in their whole, natural, unprocessed state.

- *Get spicy.* Flavor your food with herbs and spices, rather than salt. Lemon juice and vinegar also add flavor.

- *Read labels.* Look for "low sodium," "low salt," "reduced sodium," and "no salt added" on food labels.

- *Reach for low-sodium tomato products.* Tomato sauce, tomato paste, and other canned tomato products are an excellent source of potassium, as well as other important vitamins and antioxidants. But, man, are they high in sodium! Luckily, most brands offer low-sodium options.

- *Watch the condiments.* Ketchup, mustard, soy sauce, barbecue sauce, and other condiments can contain an enormous amount of sodium. Look for low-salt/low-sodium versions.

- *Make your own salsa.* Salsa from a jar often has so much salt in it. It's easy to make your own by combining chopped tomatoes, onions, jalapeño, lime juice, cilantro, and garlic. Check out my recipe for Dr. Juan's Salsa on page 211.

- *Remember that all salt has sodium.* Whether it's table salt, kosher salt, Celtic sea salt, French fleur de sel, black lava salt, or pink Himalayan salt, it all contains sodium. Although various types of salt deliver subtly different flavors, don't be fooled by the claims that gourmet salts are healthier than table salt. Sodium is sodium.

- *Check for salt in spices.* Some spice blends are really just salt with a few spices added. (Because salt is typically cheaper than spices, adding salt raises a spice mix's profit margin for its manufacturer.) For example, some types of chili powder aren't pure ground chilies, but a mix of some chili powder and a whole lot of salt. Choose salt-free chili powder—not only will you skip the salt, but you'll get stronger chili flavor too.

▪ *Think twice about buying prepared food.* Store-bought convenience foods, such as the ready-to-eat prepared foods sold in grocery stores, often contain large amounts of sodium. And because they may not come with food labels, you have no idea how much sodium you're getting.

▪ *Give 'em a rinse.* Canned beans can save you a lot of time at the stove, but some contain sodium. Toss them in a colander and rinse them with cold water, and you'll wash away much of the sodium.

▪ *Skip the processed meats.* As we discussed in chapter 6, processed meats such as sausage, bacon, ham, and luncheon meats have been linked to a higher risk of several health problems. They also tend to be loaded with sodium, which is one more reason to avoid them. Choose unprocessed chicken, seafood, pork, or beef instead—or, better yet, go with a plant-based protein such as beans, peas, lentils, or nuts.

▪ *Don't add salt to cooking water.* You may be accustomed to putting salt in the water in which you cook pasta, rice, and other grains. If you shake that habit, you'll cut down on sodium and probably won't notice any difference in taste. And keep in mind that packaged rice and grain mixes often contain large amounts of sodium—best to start out with whole grain rice and add your own spices.

▪ *Talk with your restaurant server.* Restaurant chefs are famous for the astonishing amount of salt they pour onto food. Ask your server to have your food prepared without added salt.

▪ *Take it one shake at a time.* If cutting back on salt all at once is too difficult, do it in small steps—for example, use half the amount of salt you're accustomed to using for a week or two, and then when you're accustomed to that change in taste, cut back a little more. Your taste buds will adjust to flavor changes over time, and before you know it, you'll develop a new enjoyment for the naturally delicious taste of food that in the past had been hidden under all that salt.

Potassium, magnesium, and calcium

If sodium is thought of as a bad guy in the world of high blood pressure, potassium, magnesium, and calcium are the good guys. These three minerals help relax blood vessels and lower blood pressure. Although you can get potassium, magnesium, and calcium from supplements, I believe it's best to get them from foods. Luckily, you can get ample amounts of these crucial minerals easily by eating a healthy diet—as you will when you follow the Mojito Diet.

Here's an easy way to get all three of these important minerals in one go: by eating dairy foods. Drink a glass of milk, eat a cup of yogurt, enjoy a cube of cheese, and you'll be helping your cardiovascular system by filling up on potassium, magnesium, and calcium, as well as protein. The DASH eating plan gives dairy a big thumbs-up and so do I; I encourage you to have at least two servings of dairy daily. These and other great sources of these three very useful blood pressure–lowering minerals include:

Potassium-rich foods: Acorn squash, almonds, apricots, avocados, bananas, beans (especially pinto beans, kidney beans, navy beans, white beans, and black beans), cantaloupe, chicken and turkey, citrus fruits (especially oranges), leafy greens (especially Swiss chard, beet greens, kale, and spinach), lentils and split peas, lima beans, milk, peaches, plantains, pork, seafood (especially salmon, clams, mackerel, halibut, yellowfin tuna, snapper, Pacific rockfish, and rainbow trout), sunflower seeds, sweet potatoes, tomatoes and tomato products (such as tomato paste, tomato sauce, tomato puree, and tomato juice), vegetable juice, white potatoes with their skin, yogurt, and zucchini.

Magnesium-rich foods: Avocados, bananas, beans (especially black beans and kidney beans), brown rice, chicken, edamame, fish such as salmon and halibut, fortified breakfast cereals, leafy green vegetables such as spinach, milk, nuts (especially almonds, cashews, peanuts, and their butters), oats, soy milk, white potatoes with their skin, and yogurt.

Calcium-rich foods: Dairy products (such as milk and yogurt), fish with edible bones (such as canned salmon and canned sardines), foods that are enriched with calcium (such as soy milk, tofu, and breakfast cereals), and leafy green vegetables.

As you can see, it's not difficult to include foods that are high in potassium, magnesium, and calcium in your daily eating plan, because there are so many of them to choose from. When each of your meals and snacks includes lean protein along with a fruit and/or a vegetable—as is the case in the Mojito Diet—you have the opportunity to eat blood pressure–lowering foods throughout the day. Cut back on salt, add in exercise, and you'll be taking big steps toward improving the health of your arteries and lowering your blood pressure.

And once you start losing weight, you boost your chances of improving your blood pressure even more—researchers have found that dropping just five or ten pounds can have a positive impact on the blood pressure of overweight people.

MOJITO DIET SUCCESS STORY: **YVETTE**

Feeling More Energetic

Although lowering her risk of health problems was important to Yvette when she started the Mojito Diet, her main goal was to feel more energetic. Yvette, the fifty-one-year-old vice president of a nonprofit organization, often felt sluggish during the day. However, once she started following the healthy Mojito Diet food plan, Yvette was thrilled to discover that she had more energy than she'd had for quite some time.

Yvette, who admits to a history of yo-yo dieting, found that when she followed fad diets in the past, she would lose weight quickly and gain it back almost as fast. But with the Mojito Diet, Yvette turned away from fad diets and committed to a healthy eating plan she could stick with long-term. In four months, she lost a total of twenty pounds and two inches off her waistline.

"The Mojito Diet taught me how to eat better and become more experimental with my meals to make them healthy and fun," Yvette says. "When I started the Mojito Diet, I had already lost seven pounds on my own, but did not feel as good and was usually hungry! Incorporating the Mojito Diet tips and eating plan, I added an additional steady thirteen-pound weight loss, which I've kept off."

The Mojito Diet taught Yvette a few very important lessons, such as why it's important to cut out the low-quality carbohydrates that add weight without nutrients and why it's worthwhile to weigh food for portion control. "It did not feel like a diet, because it allowed for many healthy food combinations in a controlled, portioned manner," Yvette says. "I like that I can have a drink on the weekend, to not eliminate the social aspect of living life."

Despite some initial misgivings, Yvette found she enjoyed fasting three days a week. "When I first tried fasting I wasn't sure I could do it, but Dr. Juan encouraged me not to give up," Yvette says. "I kept with it, and I soon felt that I had more energy when I worked out and was not as hungry during the day. Now it's part of my week! My advice to others is not to give up on fasting. It takes getting used to, but it drives lasting results."

PART THREE

THE MOJITO DIET GUIDELINES AND MENUS

Now that you've learned all about how to change the way you think about diet and exercise, as well as the specific foods that can fuel weight loss, it's time to start eating and drinking!

The Mojito Diet begins with the Grain Drop plan. During this first week, you'll kick weight loss into high gear by cutting out grains and focusing on protein, vegetables, fruits, nuts, seeds, and healthy fats. Grain Drop is designed to deliver quick results that will inspire and excite you.

Next you'll move on to the Clean 16 Fast plan. During this second week of the Mojito Diet, you'll add grains back in to your daily menus. And you'll also start to discover the benefits of sixteen-hour fasting by introducing three Clean 16 Fasts into your week. The Clean 16 Fast plan is designed to optimize your weight loss while making room for bread, rice, crackers, and other enjoyable grains.

Along the way, my Mojito Diet menus will show you exactly what to eat to optimize weight loss. And my delicious Latin-inspired recipes will wow you with a wide range of tasty, flavorful breakfasts, soups, salads, and main dishes.

And don't forget the mojitos! Each week you'll celebrate your success and reward yourself with fun, refreshing mojitos!

In the weeks that follow, you'll alternate week by week between Grain Drop and the Clean 16 Fast until you meet your weight-loss goal. Then, once you hit your target weight, you'll keep your weight off long-term by following the Mojito Maintenance Plan.

A Choice of Approaches

As you follow Grain Drop, the Clean 16 Fast, and the Mojito Maintenance Plan, you'll have two choices: You can use my recommended meal plans, which include recipes for delicious Latin-inspired meals, or you can use my guidelines to put together your own personalized meal plans. You can even mix and match between the two, making swaps that will lead to a customized plan that best fits your tastes and preferences. Whatever you choose, I'll make it simple for you to know exactly what to eat at each meal and snack throughout the day, every day.

Even though we'll be focusing on food, I want you to remember that exercise is also a crucial contributor to weight loss. In chapter 4, we talked about the importance of exercise for weight loss and optimal health. If you haven't started doing your salsa dancing, walking, swimming, cycling, or other enjoyable fitness activities, now's a great time to begin! These activities burn calories, which is fantastic, of course. But they also make you feel so good about yourself and help boost your motivation to follow your healthy eating plan and stay committed to meeting your goals. You don't have to set aside big chunks of time for exercise each day—just fit in ten-minute activity bursts a couple times a day. Or if ten minutes is too much, move for five minutes, and add more as you get fitter and start developing an exercise habit. Remind yourself every day that any amount of any kind of exercise is better than none at all. Get moving, my friend—you'll be happy you did!

Food Groups, Servings, and Portion Sizes

As you follow the Mojito Diet, I'll ask you to keep three main things in mind:

1. Food Groups: The foods you eat are divided into several different food groups.

Throughout the Mojito Diet, you'll eat foods in each of several food groups. These are:

- Protein (lean meats, poultry, seafood, eggs, soy, dairy, beans, peas, and lentils)
- Vegetables
- Fruit
- Grains
- Nuts and seeds
- Healthy fats
- Mojitos! (or dessert)

Each of these food groups contributes crucial nutrients to a healthy, disease-preventing diet (except for the mojitos, which are a reward). And each plays an important part in weight loss. With the exception of grains, which you will not eat during the Week 1 Grain Drop, and mojitos (or dessert), which are occasional treats, you'll eat foods from each group every day.

2. Servings: Each day you'll eat a specific number of servings from each food group.

To lose weight, it's not enough just to eat healthy foods. You must also make smart choices about the *amount* of food you eat. That's why the Mojito Diet provides a specific number of servings of various groups of food each day. Serving numbers have been carefully calibrated to provide you with enough food to help you lose weight while still feeling satisfied.

The number of servings you eat each day differs during Grain Drop, the Clean 16 Fast, and the Mojito Maintenance Plan. That's because our goals are slightly different each week.

3. *Portion Sizes*: As you get started with the Mojito Diet, you'll measure your foods to make sure you eat the right-size portions.

Eating the proper portions of various foods is very important as you try to lose weight. Most people are accustomed to estimating portion sizes by eye as they cook and serve themselves food. But studies have found that we are quite terrible at estimating portion sizes! For example, the amount of breakfast cereal that you think is one portion is more likely to be two, or even three servings, which could mean you're eating up to three times more food than you need for breakfast. No wonder the pounds keep piling on!

That's why an important part of the Mojito Diet's first weeks is to measure your food portions to ensure you're eating the right amount. You won't have to do this forever—before you know it, you'll be good at estimating portion sizes accurately. But for now, I'd like you to make sure you have measuring spoons, measuring cups, and a kitchen scale. You don't have to spend a lot on a good kitchen scale. For example, the Ozeri Pronto Digital Multifunction Kitchen and Food Scale, which has received thousands of five-star reviews on Amazon, costs less than fifteen dollars.

The Mojito Diet Food Charts starting on page 153 show you exactly what foods are in each food group and what the serving size is for each food.

Before You Get Started

Here are a few things to know before you begin following the Mojito Diet.

How much weight you lose will depend on a few different things.
Individual weight loss on the Mojito Diet varies based on how closely you follow the recommended eating plans and how much you weigh. For example, people who are obese are likely to lose more weight at a faster rate than those who are less overweight. On average, you can expect to lose two to three pounds per week while following the Mojito Diet,

although I've seen people lose as much as six pounds during their first week following the Grain Drop plan.

You have lots of flexibility. All of the meals and snacks in the daily meal plans have been carefully configured to give you the amounts and types of foods that will help you lose weight in a healthy, speedy, successful way. However, you are free to make substitutions provided you choose other foods in the same food group and the same serving size. For example, if the menu calls for a half cup of berries for breakfast, which counts as one fruit serving, and you're not in the mood for berries, go ahead and choose another fruit such as an apple or an orange instead. Simply check the Mojito Diet Food Charts (see page 153) before making your substitution to be sure you have the right amount for a single serving.

You can swap in different recipes. If you don't like the recommended recipe in a meal plan, feel free to choose another from the Recipe Guide (see page 187). Be sure to go with a recipe that is marked Grain Drop or Clean 16 Fast, depending on which week you're in, to be sure you're making the right swap.

You're welcome to drink coffee and tea. Coffee and tea can help fill you up, so go ahead and have them in moderation. However, if you add milk to your coffee or tea, choose fat-free milk. And when you're following the Clean 16 Fast, don't use milk in your coffee or tea while fasting, because only calorie-free water and Mojito Water (page 198) are recommended during fasting periods. As for sugar, it's best to leave it out of your coffee or tea. Sugar adds extra calories that really pile up. If you sweeten your coffee with two teaspoons of sugar and have three cups a day, it could lead to a weight gain of more than five pounds per year. I'm not someone who thinks sugar is an enemy that should be completely removed from your diet. However, I do think it makes sense to cut it out wherever you can, especially if you're having it in a beverage you drink several times each day. Sugar adds nothing but empty calories to your diet and can fuel your addiction to refined carbohydrates. To wean yourself off sugar in coffee or tea, start by reducing how much sugar you add, and eventually cut it out. Many of my patients have done this, and they eventually discover that their coffee or tea is just as enjoyable without sugar. Some even tell me that they like the taste better without sugar.

It's best to avoid artificial sweeteners and foods made with them, but stevia is fine. I'm okay with you using stevia, a *natural* sweetener made from an extract of the leaf of the stevia plant, which is native to South America. Stevia is two hundred times sweeter than sugar, so a little goes a long way. As for *artificial* sweeteners, I would rather you stayed away from them. An occasional diet soda is all right, but some studies have found that drinking diet soda and other artificially sweetened beverages is actually associated with weight gain, larger waist circumference, and higher rates of type 2 diabetes, high blood pressure, metabolic syndrome, and heart disease. Researchers don't really know why this association exists— maybe it's because people who use a lot of artificial sweeteners make poor dietary choices, like frequently pairing their diet soda with a burger, fries, and a deep-fried apple pie. But it's probably more complex than that. Whatever the reason, I recommend avoiding artificial sweeteners such as aspartame, sucralose, and saccharin in beverages, gelatins, frozen desserts, flans, and other foods. Instead of diet soda, reach for water, unsweetened seltzer flavored with a twist of lemon or lime, or my delicious Mojito Water (page 198). If you drink a lot of diet soda, it may seem difficult to imagine giving it up, but it's actually possible—and easier than you think—to let go of foods that don't support your good health. Do it gradually, over time, and before you know it you'll find yourself enjoying healthier choices.

Use stevia OR sugar for your mojitos. When you make your reward mojitos, it's best to make them with stevia, especially if you feel that you are addicted to sugar. Sugar is high in calories and is a source of low-quality carbohydrates. But not everyone likes stevia mojitos, and since your weekly mojitos are a reward, I want you to enjoy them! The relatively small amount of sugar in a mojito won't derail your weight-loss efforts.

You can schedule your snacks whenever you like them. My daily meal plans include an afternoon snack, because I've found that most people get hungry in the middle of the afternoon, but if you'd prefer to eat your snack at another time of day, go right ahead. Or you can split up the afternoon snack and have part of it in the morning and part of it in the afternoon. Or if you don't want a snack, you can add your snack foods to your meals. Do what works best for you. In the Mojito Diet, you can schedule your eating however you'd like. As long as you eat the recommended number of servings of each food sometime during the day and include protein and vegetables or fruit at every meal and snack, you'll be all set. The only exception is to avoid eating within two hours of bedtime, and not to eat after 8 p.m. when following the Clean 16 Fast.

Meal plans include nuts, but you don't have to eat them. Nuts play an important role in the Mojito Diet because they are high in protein, high in fiber, and a good source of several vitamins and minerals. Plus, many studies have found associations between nuts and weight loss as well as heart health. Unfortunately, nuts cause allergic reactions in some people. If you are unable to eat nuts but you can tolerate seeds, consider having them instead. However, if you're allergic to seeds as well — or if you just don't like nuts — I recommend substituting one serving of lean protein for a serving of nuts. Pair it with vegetables, and you'll have a full package of protein and fiber — for example, a piece of cheese and some carrots, or hummus and red peppers. That way you'll be getting fiber, protein, and other nutrients.

Vegetables are unlimited! In every part of the Mojito Diet — Grain Drop, the Clean 16 Fast, and the Mojito Maintenance Plan — you can eat as many vegetables as you like! The only exceptions to this rule are potatoes and sweet potatoes. Since these are higher in calories than most other vegetables, limit potatoes of any kind to one serving per day. But otherwise, there's no limit on vegetables. And remember, Dr. Juan's Salsa (page 211) is 100 percent vegetables, so you can have as much of it as you want. I like to use it as a dip for raw vegetables such as baby carrots, bell pepper strips, and celery sticks.

Starchy produce is okay with me. Some diets don't allow, or severely limit, starchy vegetables (such as potatoes, sweet potatoes, carrots, corn, green peas, plantains, and squash), starchy fruits (such as bananas), and high-sugar fruits (such as pineapple and papaya). But the Mojito Diet makes room for these delicious, nutritious foods. They provide important nutrients including antioxidants, blood pressure–lowering potassium and magnesium, and other vitamins and minerals. Their fiber content helps offset any impact they may have on blood sugar. My only limitation is to keep potatoes and sweet potatoes to one serving per day. If you have diabetes, follow the recommendations from your doctor or diabetes educator regarding your intake of fruits and starchy vegetables.

An occasional serving of chips is okay. Overall I'd rather you avoid foods like tortilla chips, because they add no nutrients to your diet. As you cut back on foods in an effort to lose weight, it's best to focus on nutritious foods rather than high-calorie snacks. However, if you've got a craving for tortilla chips that just won't stop, have a 1-ounce serving of whole grain chips, count it as a grain, and throw the rest of the chips in the bag away so you don't eat them later.

Recipe swaps are okay. If you see an ingredient that you don't like in one of my recipes, go ahead and swap in another similar ingredient. Just make sure you choose a substitute ingredient in the same serving size from the same food group—use the Mojito Diet Food Charts (see page 153) to guide you. For example, if a recipe calls for fish and you'd rather use shrimp or chicken or lean pork, you are welcome to make that change. The Mojito Diet is designed to offer you maximum flexibility within a structure that optimizes weight loss and health.

You can have other drinks too. Mojitos are delicious—I've included recipes for many different types in the Recipe Guide (see page 187). But you can have other types of alcoholic beverages instead—perhaps a different kind of mixed drink, or one serving of beer or wine. When having mixed drinks, choose lower-calorie mixers such as seltzer, stevia, and 100 percent fruit juices. You can have your reward mojito at any time, with two exceptions: Don't break your Clean 16 Fast with a mojito at lunch, and don't have it after 8 p.m. the night before you begin a Clean 16 Fast.

Or, you can have dessert. If you choose to have a dessert rather than a reward mojito, be sure to choose the right serving size. A serving of dessert is one small slice of cake, one or two cookies, one small serving of flan, or other sweets or treats with up to 200 calories.

It's up to you and your doctor to decide whether to take a multivita-min. The Mojito Diet is very nutritious, and if you follow it as written you should get the nutrients you need. Talk with your doctor about whether you should take multivitamins or other supplements.

My recipes are (mostly) low in salt. In chapter 9, we talked about the link between salt and high blood pressure, and I recommended cutting down on salt in foods whether or not you have high blood pressure. For this reason, most of my recipes are low in salt, and I recommend unsalted foods such as unsalted nuts. However, a few of my recipes do contain salt or salty foods, such as pickles or capers. Why? Because a little taste of salt really makes those recipes shine. Although it's great to cut down on salt, you don't have to eliminate it completely unless you have high blood pressure. In the few recipes that include salt or salty ingredients, feel free to make your own decision about whether to use it based on your doctor's recommendations.

It's okay to substitute protein bars for a meal or snack—but only occasionally. When you're on the run, eating a protein bar is easier than having a meal. However, although protein bars do provide protein and some other nutrients, they have two drawbacks: First, some are high in sugar and calories, and are more like protein-enriched candy bars than healthy foods. Second, even if they are pumped up with nutrients, they're still not as good for you as whole foods. My advice is to choose protein bars that are low in sugar, and to eat them only when necessary.

I recommend fat-free milk and yogurt. You'll notice that the Mojito Diet calls for fat-free or low-fat milk, yogurt, and soft cheeses. I've made this choice because fat-free and low-fat dairy foods are considerably lower in calories and saturated fat than their full-fat counterparts. We don't count calories in the Mojito Diet, but we do try to avoid excess calories to move you to your weight-loss goals in the most efficient way. If you really prefer full-fat milk, yogurt, and fresh cheeses, you can make that choice, but doing so may slow down your weight loss.

The exception to this is some types of hard cheese, such as cheddar, Parmesan, Swiss, mozzarella, and Jack cheeses. Although fat-free and low-fat hard cheeses are available, I find that most of them don't taste very good and they don't tend to melt well in recipes. So I make room for full-fat hard cheese in the Mojito Diet. My view is that it's better to eat slightly smaller amounts of full-fat hard cheese than larger portions of inferior-tasting cheese. But if you have found low-fat or fat-free varieties of hard cheese you enjoy, choose those and you'll save some calories and saturated fat.

It's okay to swap other foods for milk. Milk and other dairy foods are included in some of my recipes and meal plans. Milk is an excellent source of blood pressure–lowering minerals such as calcium, magnesium, and potassium, and an important part of the DASH diet. However, if you don't like it or can't drink it because of allergies or intolerance, you may substitute soy milk, almond milk, or a serving of any other kind of dairy food or protein. If you opt for nondairy milks, choose varieties that are fortified with calcium and vitamin D, and choose nut milks fortified with protein.

You don't need to add protein powder to your smoothies. Unless you work out vigorously, you probably don't need the large amounts of extra protein provided by protein powders. If you follow the Mojito Diet meal plans, you should get all the protein you need to optimize weight loss.

DR. JUAN'S WISDOM

EATING OUT ON THE MOJITO DIET

Most Americans eat out at least once a week, and some of us find ourselves having meals away from home much more often than that. Although it's easier to follow the Mojito Diet with home-prepared meals, eating at restaurants is part of life, and I don't want you to have to give up this enjoyable, convenient option just because you're trying to lose weight and improve your health. I do recommend that you prepare your food at home as often as possible, because doing so gives you the most control over what you eat, but I don't expect you to be a slave to your kitchen. Keep a few guidelines in mind and you can stay mostly within the parameters of the plan.

When you're eating in restaurants, think of two things: protein and produce. Let's start with the protein. Go for "naked protein," which is lean meat, poultry, and seafood without breading, sauces, or toppings. As for produce, I'm referring to veggies, salad, or fruit. You can find naked protein and produce on menus in one form or another at almost any restaurant. For example:

▶ Grilled salmon with sautéed vegetables at a high-end restaurant

▶ A Caesar salad (hold the croutons) topped with grilled chicken or shrimp at a fast-casual place

▶ A burrito bowl with naked chicken, black beans, and lettuce (hold the rice) at a Tex-Mex restaurant

▶ Yellowtail and king crab with fresh greens at a sushi place

▶ A burger without the bun plus a side salad at a fast-food restaurant

▶ A veggie omelet with a side of fresh fruit salad at a diner

▶ Yogurt or cheese and a banana at an airport newsstand

If you have salad, ask for the dressing on the side and try to estimate a serving size of about a tablespoon. Healthy fats such as avocado or guacamole are fine, but remember that calories add up fast with fats, and the amount your server gives you will probably be far more than a single serving. As for the serving size of the naked protein, eat an amount that looks like it's about equal to the size of a deck of cards (4 ounces of protein) and either take home what's left or just leave it on the plate.

If you're in a restaurant where the naked protein and produce guidelines simply won't work—for example, if every choice is breaded or smothered in sauce—focus instead on the *amount* of food you're eating. Most restaurant meals provide two to four times more food than you need, so try to eat only a quarter or half of the meal and leave the rest. And if it's impossible to avoid eating grains on Grain Drop days—perhaps you're having dinner with your kids and another family, and pizza is the only food on offer—go ahead and have a slice, but skip the thick edge of the crust. Fill out your meal with a green salad. You do want to stay on your plan, but you don't have to be neurotic about it. If you must go off-plan for a meal, try as best you can to make good choices and then get back on the plan at your next meal or snack. The goal is not to be perfect all the time, but to do your best while continuing to enjoy your life.

Finally, if you eat out a lot, spend some time identifying the restaurants that are best able to accommodate your needs. Some are very willing to work with diners to create a meal that fits their dietary requirements, and others aren't. And if you dine out often with friends and coworkers, talk with them about your weight-loss goals and steer them toward restaurants that have protein and produce options that fit into your plan.

Now You're Ready to Eat

In the next section, I'll tell you all about my Week 1 Grain Drop plan. Then I'll show you my Week 2 Clean 16 Fast. Finally, I'll share my Mojito Maintenance Plan. I can't wait for you to start eating and losing!

The Mojito Diet at a Glance

WEEK 1: Grain Drop

- No grains! Cut out all breads, rice, pasta, tortillas, and other grains for one week.

- Eat high-protein foods and high-fiber fruits and vegetables at every meal and snack, plus healthy fats.

- Measure your food to learn about healthy portion sizes.

- Reward yourself with two mojitos!

- Drink plenty of water or make my special Mojito Water (page 198).

WEEK 2: Clean 16 Fast

- Do three nonconsecutive days of sixteen-hour fasts by skipping breakfast three days of the week. (Be sure to finish your last meal before 8 p.m. the night before.)

- On the Clean 16 Fast days, eat a regular lunch and dinner.

- Eat grains again! Have two to three servings of whole grains each day.

- Continue to eat high-protein foods, healthy fats, and high-fiber fruits and vegetables at every meal.

- Don't make up for skipped breakfast by eating more at lunch, snack, or dinner.

- Continue to drink Mojito Water (page 198) while you fast to fill up and flush out toxins.

- Reward yourself with two mojitos!

WEEK 3: Repeat Grain Drop

WEEK 4: Repeat Clean 16 Fast

After that: Continue cycling through the Grain Drop and the Clean 16 Fast, week by week, until you reach your goal weight. Then move on to the Mojito Maintenance Plan.

THE MOJITO MAINTENANCE PLAN:

- Eat a healthy diet five days a week.

- Follow the Grain Drop plan one day a week.

- Follow the Clean 16 Fast and skip breakfast one day a week.

- Add extra Grain Drop days if you start to regain lost weight.

- Reward yourself with three mojitos!

The Mojito Diet Food Charts

Protein

Includes lean meats, poultry, seafood, eggs, soy, dairy, beans (adzuki beans, black beans, great northern beans, kidney beans, pinto beans, red beans, white beans, etc.), peas (such as split peas, black-eyed peas/cowpeas, chickpeas, pigeon peas), and lentils

FOOD	SERVING SIZE	NOTES
Lean meats (such as lean cuts of beef, pork, and lamb)	1 ounce cooked (or 1 ¼ ounces raw)	Beef: Choose leanest cuts, such as eye of round, tenderloin filet, and sirloin
		Pork: Choose leanest cuts, such as pork tenderloin, lean pork chops, and top loin pork roast
		Remove all visible fat
Poultry	1 ounce cooked (or 1 ¼ ounces raw)	Choose white meat with skin removed
Seafood (fish and shellfish)	1 ounce cooked (or 1 ¼ ounces raw)	Aim for at least 8 ounces per week
Canned tuna, salmon, or chicken	1 ounce after draining	Choose varieties packed in water, without added salt
Eggs	1 whole egg or 3 egg whites	
Soy (tofu and tempeh)	1 ounce	
Milk	1 cup	Choose fat-free or low-fat
Buttermilk	1 cup	Choose fat-free or low-fat
Soy milk	1 cup	Choose fat-free or low-fat varieties fortified with calcium and vitamin D and without added sweeteners
Nut milk, such as almond milk	1 cup	Choose varieties fortified with protein, calcium, and vitamin D and without added sweeteners
Yogurt (regular, Greek, or Icelandic)	1 single-serve container (5 to 8 ounces)	Choose fat-free or low-fat yogurts without added sweeteners or mix-ins

FOOD	SERVING SIZE	NOTES
Kefir (cultured milk drink)	8 ounces	Choose fat-free or low-fat
Hard cheese (such as cheddar, Parmesan, mozzarella, Gouda, Swiss, Monterey Jack, cotija, Pepper Jack, Manchego, etc.)	1 ounce (about ¼ cup if shredded or grated)	Choose low-fat varieties if you like the way they taste; otherwise, choose full-fat hard cheeses
Soft cheese (such as cottage cheese, ricotta, feta, Queso Blanco, Queso Fresco, Panela, etc.)	½ cup	Choose low-fat varieties; avoid unpasteurized cheeses, because they can cause food poisoning; pregnant women and anyone with a compromised immune system should eat only pasteurized cheeses
Cooked or canned beans, peas, lentils, or lima beans	½ cup	Choose low-sodium varieties and rinse canned legumes to remove sodium
Hummus	3 tablespoons	
Protein powder	⅓ scoop (1 scoop = 3 servings of protein)	Choose varieties without added sugar; unless you exercise vigorously you probably don't need to add protein powder to your meals
Protein bars	¼ bar (1 bar = 4 servings of protein)	Choose bars that are low in sugar; use as meal replacements only occasionally, because it's better to eat whole foods

Vegetables

Includes bean sprouts, bell peppers (green, red, orange, yellow), broccoli, cabbage, carrots, cauliflower, celery, collard greens, corn, cucumbers, endive, escarole, green beans, green peas, hearts of palm, jícama, kale, lettuce, mushrooms, mustard greens, onions, pumpkin, roasted red peppers (in water), romaine, spinach, squash (acorn, butternut, summer, winter), sweet potatoes, tomatillos, tomatoes, turnip greens, watercress, wax beans, white potatoes, and zucchini

FOOD	SERVING SIZE	NOTES
Raw leafy vegetables	1 cup	Choose plenty of dark leafy greens, which are rich sources of nutrients
Chopped raw vegetables	½ cup	Choose a rainbow of vegetables, including yellow, orange, red, green, and purple
Cooked vegetables	½ cup	If using frozen or canned, choose "naked" varieties without added salt, sugar, or sauces
Vegetable juice (tomato or mixed vegetable)	¾ cup (6 ounces)	Choose low-sodium varieties
White potatoes	½ cup cooked, or ½ small baked potato	Limit to no more than 1 serving per day of potatoes of any kind
Sweet potatoes	½ cup cooked, or ½ small baked sweet potato	Limit to no more than 1 serving per day of potatoes of any kind

Fruit

Includes apples, bananas, blackberries, blueberries, cantaloupe, clementines, fruit salad, grapefruit, grapes, kiwi, oranges and other citrus fruits, peaches, pears, pineapple, plantains, plums, raspberries, strawberries, and watermelon

FOOD	SERVING SIZE	NOTES
Whole fruit	1 small fruit or ½ medium or large fruit	Choose a wide variety of fruits
Chopped fruit or small whole fruit, such as berries	½ cup	Choose a rainbow of fruits to get a range of nutrients and antioxidants
Frozen fruit	½ cup	Choose varieties with no added sugar
Canned fruit	½ cup	Choose varieties with no added sugar or syrups
Fruit juice, unsweetened	½ cup	Limit to no more than 1 serving per day or less because fruit juice is high in sugar and low in fiber
Plantains	½ medium plantain	Eat only occasionally, because plantains are high in calories
Dried fruit	¼ cup	Limit to no more than 1 serving per day or less because dried fruit is high in sugar

Nuts and Seeds

Includes almonds, almond butter, cashews, cashew butter, hazelnuts, pea-nuts, peanut butter, pistachios, walnuts, pumpkin seeds, sesame seeds, and sunflower seeds

FOOD	SERVING SIZE	NOTES
Nuts	1 ounce (approximately 2 tablespoons)	Choose unsalted nuts without added sugar or sweeteners
Nut butter	2 tablespoons	Choose unsalted or low-sodium nut butter
Seeds	2 tablespoons	Choose unsalted seeds

Healthy Fats

Includes healthy oils, salad dressings, olives, avocado, guacamole, and tahini

FOOD	SERVING SIZE	NOTES
Healthy oils (canola, corn, flaxseed, grapeseed, olive, peanut, safflower, sesame, soybean)	1 tablespoon	Because fats are high in calories, be sure to measure carefully to avoid using too much
Full-fat salad dressing	1 tablespoon	Measure carefully
Low-fat or fat-free salad dressing	2 tablespoons	
Olives (black or green)	20 small or 10 large olives	
Avocado	½ small or ¼ medium avocado	
Guacamole	¼ cup	Measure carefully
Tahini	1 tablespoon	
Butter	1 teaspoon	Because of its high saturated fat content, butter is not considered a healthy fat, so the portion size is much smaller than that of healthier fats
Light coconut milk	½ cup	Although coconut milk is high in saturated fat (even "light" varieties), it's an irreplaceable ingredient in some Latin recipes; use it only occasionally, and be sure to choose light/low-fat versions

Grains*

Breads, cereal, granola, whole grains, rice, pasta, popcorn, and snack chips

FOOD	SERVING SIZE	NOTES
Whole grain bread	1 slice	Choose brands with a whole grain listed as the first ingredient on the nutrition label
Ready-to-eat cereal	1 ounce, or between ½ cup and 1¼ cups, depending on the type of cereal	Choose whole grain varieties with at least 4 grams of fiber per serving
Oatmeal and cooked cereal, unsweetened	½ cup cooked	Choose unsweetened varieties
Granola, low-sugar or unsweetened	¼ cup	Choose varieties that are lower in sugar and fat
Whole grains (such as amaranth, barley, bulgur, quinoa)	½ cup cooked (¼ cup uncooked)	Cook them yourself or buy precooked frozen grains with no added salt, seasonings, or sauces
Rice, brown	½ cup cooked (¼ cup uncooked)	Choose brown rice
Pasta, whole grain	½ cup cooked (1 ounce uncooked)	Choose whole grain pasta
Bagel, whole grain	1 mini bagel	Choose whole grain bagels
Tortilla, whole grain	6-inch tortilla	Choose corn or whole grain flour varieties
Popcorn, air-popped	3 cups	Choose plain, air-popped varieties without salt
English muffin, whole grain	½ muffin	Choose whole grain varieties
Crackers, whole grain	1 ounce	Choose whole grain and/or seed-based varieties, preferably low-salt
Snack chips, whole grain	1 ounce	Choose whole grain and/or seed-based varieties, preferably low-salt
Roll, whole grain	1 ounce	Choose whole grain varieties

Although grains are not included in the Grain Drop phase, you will add them during the Clean 16 Fast week and the Mojito Maintenance Plan.

WEEK 1:
The Grain Drop Plan

Welcome to Week 1 of the Mojito Diet! The Week 1 Grain Drop plan is designed to kick-start your weight loss and start delivering fast results that will inspire you to stay committed to healthier eating and permanent weight loss.

During these first seven days, I will ask you to do something that might seem a bit difficult at first: to give up all grain-based foods such as bread, rice, tortillas, pasta, crackers, and cereal. I know that may sound tough, but believe me, it's a worthwhile step that will bring you big rewards. And don't worry—you can start eating these grain-based foods again next week.

Remember, the Mojito Diet eating plans are built around three important guidelines:

1. *You'll eat foods from a variety of food groups each day.* The Mojito Diet Food Charts starting on page 153 show you exactly which foods are in each food group.

2. *You'll measure your foods to make sure you eat the right-size portions.* The Mojito Diet Food Charts also show you portion sizes for every food.

3. *You'll eat a specific number of servings from each food group.* The chart below shows how many daily servings of each food to aim for this week.

GRAIN DROP DAILY SERVINGS

FOOD GROUP	DAILY SERVINGS
Protein (lean meats, poultry, seafood, eggs, soy, dairy, beans/peas/lentils)	8 to 10*
Vegetables	5 or more
Fruit	3
Nuts/seeds	1
Healthy fats	2 to 3*
Mojitos!	2 per week

Eat fewer servings for faster weight loss.

Follow my plan, or create your own

As you do the Grain Drop plan this week, you have the choice of following my meal plan, which includes lots of fabulous recipes, or creating your own. And if you follow my plan, you have the option of swapping in other foods—just use the Mojito Diet Food Charts (see page 153) to create your own meal. I've provided plenty of recipes for foods that fit right into Grain Drop and the Clean 16 Fast, but don't feel that you have to use them all—I know schedules are tight, and we don't always have time to cook meals from scratch. But I've made it easy for you to do whatever works best for you.

For example, at breakfast on Day 1, the Grain Drop meal plan recommends the Any Fruit Parfait (you'll find a recipe for this enjoyable breakfast in the recipe section). But if you don't feel like having the Any Fruit Parfait, feel free to swap in your own breakfast choice made with two servings of protein and two servings of fruit. The Mojito Diet Food Charts show you all the choices you have for those protein and fruit servings, along with serving sizes.

You can also design your own Grain Drop meal plan. Use the instructions starting on page 168.

The Grain Drop Plan

I hope you're hungry, because it's time to start eating. The following meal plan has my suggested food choices and a detailed menu for every day this week, along with the number of food servings each meal provides. You'll also find a planning guide you can use to design your own Grain Drop plan for Week 1. Recipes can be found in the Recipe Guide starting on page 187. I recommend beginning your meal plan on Sunday, but if you'd rather start on a different day of the week, go right ahead.

WEEK 1, DAY 1
Sunday

. . . .

Breakfast

Any Fruit Parfait (page 200) made with tropical fruits (mango, banana, pineapple) and ginger

▶ *Or your choice of any 2 servings protein and 2 servings fruit*

Lunch

Latin Chicken Salad (page 205)

1 apple

▶ *Or your choice of any 4 servings protein, 2 servings (or more) vegetables, 1 serving fruit, and 1 serving healthy fats*

Afternoon Snack

½ cup (or more) baby carrots

1 ounce almonds

▶ *Or your choice of any 1 serving (or more) vegetables and 1 serving nuts/seeds*

Dinner

Seared Steak Chimichurri (page 219)

2 cups spinach sautéed in ½ tablespoon olive oil

▶ *Or your choice of any 4 servings protein, 2 servings (or more) vegetables, and 1 to 2 servings healthy fats*

WEEK 1, DAY 2
Monday

. . . .

Breakfast

1 cup blueberries

Any Veggie Egg Scramble (page 201) made Mexican-style, with red onions, green bell peppers, tomatoes, cilantro, and chili powder

▶ *Or your choice of any 2 servings protein and 2 servings fruit*

Lunch

Gazpacho with Pinto Beans and Avocado (page 212)

1 cup fat-free milk

1 small banana

▶ *Or your choice of any 4 servings protein, 2 servings (or more) vegetables, 1 serving fruit, and 1 serving healthy fats*

Afternoon Snack

½ cup (or more) sliced red bell peppers

1 ounce pistachios

▶ *Or your choice of any 1 serving (or more) vegetables and 1 serving nuts/seeds*

Dinner

Pork Tenderloin with Warm Salsa Verde (page 220)

½ small baked sweet potato

▶ *Or your choice of any 4 servings protein, 2 servings (or more) vegetables, and 1 to 2 servings healthy fats*

WEEK 1, DAY 3
Tuesday

. . . .

Breakfast

Any Fruit Smoothie (page 202) made with mixed berries (blueberries, raspberries, and blackberries)

▶ *Or your choice of any 2 servings protein and 2 servings fruit*

Lunch

Mexican Black Bean Soup (page 213)

1 cup fat-free milk

½ cup melon

▶ *Or your choice of any 4 servings protein, 2 servings (or more) vegetables, 1 serving fruit, and 1 serving healthy fats*

Afternoon Snack

½ cup (or more) baby carrots

1 ounce walnuts

▶ *Or your choice of any 1 serving (or more) vegetables and 1 serving nuts/seeds*

Dinner

Mojito Salmon (page 221)

Tossed side salad made with 2 cups spinach, sliced red onion, and 1 tablespoon salad dressing

▶ *Or your choice of any 4 servings protein, 2 servings (or more) vegetables, and 1 to 2 servings healthy fats*

WEEK 1, DAY 4
Wednesday

Breakfast

Any Fruit Salad with Fresh Cheese (page 203) made with bananas, cinnamon, and cottage cheese

▶ *Or your choice of any 2 servings protein and 2 servings fruit*

Lunch

Spanish Veggie Salad with Tuna and Potatoes (page 206)

1 orange

▶ *Or your choice of any 4 servings protein, 2 servings (or more) vegetables, 1 serving fruit, and 1 serving healthy fats*

Afternoon Snack

2 tablespoons almond butter spread on 2 large celery stalks

▶ *Or your choice of any 1 serving (or more) vegetables and 1 serving nuts/seeds*

Dinner

Chicken Cutlets with Sherry Mushrooms (page 222)

½ small baked sweet potato

▶ *Or your choice of any 4 servings protein, 2 servings (or more) vegetables, and 1 to 2 servings healthy fats*

WEEK 1, DAY 5

Thursday

. . . .

Breakfast

1 cup chopped mango

Family Breakfast Bake (page 203)

▶ *Or your choice of any 2 servings protein and 2 servings fruit*

Lunch

Hearty Tomato Salad with Black Beans (page 207)

1 small banana

▶ *Or your choice of any 4 servings protein, 2 servings (or more) vegetables, 1 serving fruit, and 1 serving healthy fats*

Afternoon Snack

6 ounces low-salt vegetable juice

1 ounce almonds

▶ *Or your choice of any 1 serving (or more) vegetables and 1 serving nuts/seeds*

Dinner

Brazilian Seafood Stew (page 223)

Tossed side salad made with 2 cups romaine lettuce, ¼ cup chopped green bell pepper, and 1 tablespoon salad dressing

▶ *Or your choice of any 4 servings protein, 2 servings (or more) vegetables, and 1 to 2 servings healthy fats*

WEEK 1, DAY 6
Friday (Mojito Day)

Breakfast

Any Fruit Parfait (page 200) made with mixed berries (blueberries, raspberries, and strawberries)

▶ *Or your choice of any 2 servings protein and 2 servings fruit*

Lunch

Caribbean Pumpkin Soup with Chickpeas (page 214)

1 cup fat-free milk

1 apple

▶ *Or your choice of any 4 servings protein, 2 servings (or more) vegetables, 1 serving fruit, and 1 serving healthy fats*

Afternoon Snack

½ cup (or more) celery sticks dipped in Dr. Juan's Salsa (page 211)

1 ounce peanuts

▶ *Or your choice of any 1 serving (or more) vegetables and 1 serving nuts/seeds*

Dinner

Smothered Flank Steak (page 224)

Tossed side salad made with 2 cups spring greens, ½ cup grape tomatoes, and 1 tablespoon salad dressing

▶ *Or your choice of any 4 servings protein, 2 servings (or more) vegetables, and 1 to 2 servings healthy fats*

Reward: 1 mojito! OR 1 other alcoholic beverage OR 1 serving of dessert

WEEK 1, DAY 7

Saturday (Mojito Day)

· ·

Breakfast

1 cup mixed berries

Any Veggie Egg Scramble (page 201) made with high-potassium veggies (spinach, tomatoes, and zucchini)

▶ *Or your choice of any 2 servings protein and 2 servings fruit*

Lunch

Cactus Paddle Salad (page 207)

1 cup fat-free milk

½ cup strawberries

▶ *Or your choice of any 4 servings protein, 2 servings (or more) vegetables, 1 serving fruit, and 1 serving healthy fats*

Afternoon Snack

½ cup (or more) red pepper slices

2 tablespoons peanuts

▶ *Or your choice of any 1 serving (or more) vegetables and 1 serving nuts/seeds*

Dinner

Shrimp Veracruz over Cauliflower Rice (page 225)

½ small baked sweet potato

▶ *Or your choice of any 4 servings protein, 2 servings (or more) vegetables, and 1 to 2 servings healthy fats*

Reward: 1 mojito! OR 1 other alcoholic beverage OR 1 serving of dessert

Design your own Grain Drop plan

Some people love having a meal plan all figured out for them, like the one on the previous pages. But others prefer to create their own meal plan using the foods they like best. You can do whichever you like—follow my plan or design your own using my Mojito Diet guidelines. Either way, you can eat happily on the Mojito Diet.

To create your own plan, use the serving guidelines and the Mojito Diet Food Charts starting on page 153. Choose what you'd like to eat for breakfast, lunch, dinner, and snacks, remembering not to go over the recommended daily limit. Be sure you're familiar with portion sizes and the types of foods included in each food group.

In my meal plan, your daily allotment of food is arranged into three meals and one snack. You are welcome to use this arrangement or make changes that suit your preferences. Perhaps you would rather have three larger meals and no snacks. Or maybe you'd prefer five small meals distributed throughout the day. Those are all good choices, although it's best to avoid eating within two hours of bedtime, especially if you experience heartburn or reflux. And be sure to have protein and fiber at each meal and snack, because combining the two is the best way to fill you up and get you to the next meal or snack without getting hungry. Otherwise, as long as you end up eating the recommended number of servings from each of the food groups every day, you'll get the nutrients you need and pave the way for successful weight loss.

During the day, as you follow your custom plan, be sure to measure your portions, to ensure that you don't eat too much or too little. You can even measure out your foods the night before, to save time during the day.

Use this chart to make sure you eat the right number of servings from each food group this week:

GRAIN DROP DAILY SERVINGS

FOOD GROUP	DAILY SERVINGS
Protein (lean meats, poultry, seafood, eggs, soy, dairy, beans/peas/lentils)	8 to 10
Vegetables	5 or more
Fruit	3
Nuts/seeds	1
Healthy fats	2 to 3
Mojitos!	2 per week

Here is a sample of just one way you could choose to plan a day of Week 1 meals:

WEEK 1 CUSTOM MEAL PLAN SAMPLE

BREAKFAST	LUNCH
Fruit: 2 servings Protein: 2 servings	Protein: 4 servings Vegetables: 2 or more servings Healthy fats: 1 serving Fruit: 1 serving
AFTERNOON SNACK	**DINNER**
Vegetables: 1 or more servings Nuts/seeds: 1 serving	Protein: 4 servings Vegetables: 2 or more servings Healthy fats: 1 to 2 servings

ON MOJITO DAYS (FRIDAY AND SATURDAY): 1 mojito! OR 1 mixed drink OR 1 serving of beer or wine OR 1 serving of dessert

WEEK 2:
The Clean 16 Fast Plan

Congratulations! You have completed Week 1 of the Mojito Diet and are now ready to move on to Week 2. This week, you'll start incorporating sixteen-hour fasting into your meal plan with my Clean 16 Fast. You'll do three nonconsecutive days of sixteen-hour fasts. Doing a Clean 16 Fast is quite simple. Just follow these steps:

▪ Finish your dinner the night before your fasting day by 8 p.m., and don't eat anything for the remainder of the evening.

▪ When you wake up the next morning, skip breakfast and eat nothing until lunch at noon.

▪ When you end your fast, eat the same-size lunch, afternoon snack, and dinner that you would usually eat. Do not make up for your skipped breakfast by adding more food later in the day.

▪ While you're fasting, you can drink noncaloric liquids: water, plain coffee, black tea, or green tea (with no sweetener or milk). You can also make a big pitcher of my Mojito Water (page 198) and drink it in the evening and morning. Not only does it help fill you up and prevent hunger, but it helps flush toxins from your body. Why drink Mojito Water rather than plain water? Both mint and lime are believed to have appetite-suppressing properties. And mint is a source of antioxidants that can help protect your cells from oxidative damage. But perhaps the best reason of all is that when you're drinking Mojito Water, you are less likely to feel deprived while fasting. Enjoy it cold in an attractive glass with ice, or pour it in a mug and warm it up in the microwave if you're feeling chilly. And don't drink it just when you're fasting—Mojito Water is an enjoyable treat anytime!

▪ I recommend doing three Clean 16 Fasts this week, because that's a number that works well for many people. But if you'd rather do two or four fasts per week, that's fine too.

For an in-depth look at how fasting can help with weight loss and overall health, be sure to read chapter 8.

Grains are back!

This week, you'll add bread and other grains back into your daily meal plan. You'll have two daily servings of grains on Clean 16 Fast days, and three servings on nonfasting days.

Giving up grains last week helped kick-start your weight loss by reducing your reliance on carbohydrates—especially white carbs such as white bread, white rice, and white flour tortillas. Now that you've spent a week taking a break from grains, you can start adding them back into your diet in a healthier way.

As you reintroduce grains to your diet, you'll be eating healthy whole grains such as whole grain bread, corn and whole grain tortillas, brown rice, and other whole grains. These healthy, fiber-rich grains help fill you up while supporting your digestive system.

As in Week 1, you will continue to eat satisfying amounts of lean protein, heart-healthy fats, and filling, high-fiber vegetables, fruits, legumes, and nuts. You'll also have a range of delicious foods at every meal and snack, including all kinds of amazing Latin-inspired meals that fit perfectly into your daily eating plan. And, like last week, you'll have two mojitos or desserts to look forward to!

Mojito Diet Clean 16 Fast guidelines

Like the Grain Drop plan, the Clean 16 Fast plan is built around three important guidelines:

1. You'll eat foods from a variety of food groups each day. The Mojito Diet Food Charts starting on page 153 show you exactly which foods are in each food group.

2. You'll measure foods to make sure you eat the right-size portions. The Mojito Diet Food Charts also show you portion sizes for every food.

3. You'll eat a specific number of servings from each food group. The chart below shows how many daily servings of each food to shoot for this week. Remember, on Clean 16 Fast days you'll eat fewer total servings of food than on nonfasting days. (On Clean 16 Fast days, you'll eat two fewer servings of protein, one less fruit, and one less grain than on nonfasting days. But you'll eat the same number of servings of vegetables, nuts/seeds, and healthy fats.)

CLEAN 16 FAST DAILY SERVINGS

FOOD GROUP	DAILY SERVINGS ON CLEAN 16 FAST DAYS	DAILY SERVINGS ON NONFASTING DAYS
Protein (lean meats, poultry, seafood, eggs, soy, dairy, beans/peas/lentils)	6 to 8*	8 to 10*
Vegetables	5 or more	5 or more
Fruit	2	3
Grains	2	3
Nuts/Seeds	1	1
Healthy Fats	2 to 3*	2 to 3*
Mojitos!	2 per week	2 per week

*Eat fewer servings for faster weight loss.

DR. JUAN'S WISDOM

FASTING FAQS

Q: *I don't like skipping breakfast. Do I have to do it?*

A: Of course not! But I do encourage you to give it a try. As we discussed in chapter 8, sixteen-hour fasting can deliver some great benefits for weight loss and overall health. Try it a few times, and if you really don't like it, you don't have to do it.

Q: *Will I eat less food on Clean 16 Fast days, or will I eat the same amount as on other days?*

A: On Clean 16 Fast days you'll eat less food, because you'll skip breakfast. Be sure not to eat extra food during the day, or you'll miss out on the weight-loss benefits of the fast.

Q: *I'd like to try fasting for a longer period of time—perhaps twenty hours or twenty-four hours. Is that a good idea?*

A: I consider sixteen-hour fasts to be the most effective for weight loss. If you experiment with other kinds of fasting, be sure you're still getting all of the nutritious foods your body needs.

Q: *Can I do morning exercise on Clean 16 Fast days?*

A: As long as you don't feel weak while you're exercising, it's fine to work out in the morning on Clean 16 Fast days. Some people actually prefer to exercise on an empty stomach, because they feel more focused mentally and less sluggish physically. However, if it doesn't agree with you to exercise before eating, plan to exercise later in the day, or save your morning workouts for nonfasting days. And, of course, if your doctor has told you to eat before exercising because of hypoglycemia or other health concerns, follow that advice.

Q: *Can I do Clean 16 Fasts if I have diabetes or if I'm taking insulin or other diabetes medication?*

A: I'll leave this question up to your doctor. For more on fasting, see chapter 8.

The Clean 16 Fast Plan

Once again, I recommend starting your meal plan on Sunday. But of course, if you'd rather begin on a different day, you're welcome to.

I've designated Monday, Wednesday, and Friday as your Clean 16 Fast days; all others are nonfasting days. But you can opt to do your fasts on other days if you'd prefer. Friday and Saturday are your mojito reward days.

WEEK 2, DAY 1

Sunday

....

Breakfast

Any Fruit Parfait (page 200) made with banana and mango; topped with granola

▸ *Or your choice of any 2 servings protein, 2 servings fruit, and 1 serving grains*

Lunch

The Whatever Salad Bowl (page 209) made with optional grains

½ cup blueberries

▸ *Or your choice of any 4 servings protein, 2 servings (or more) vegetables, 1 serving fruit, 1 serving grains, and 1 serving healthy fats*

Afternoon Snack

½ cup (or more) baby carrots dipped in 2 tablespoons almond butter

▸ *Or your choice of any 1 serving (or more) vegetables and 1 serving nuts/seeds*

Dinner

Open-Face Pork Tacos with Spicy Pineapple Slaw (page 226)

½ small baked sweet potato

Or your choice of any 4 servings protein, 2 servings (or more) vegetables, 1 serving grains, and 1 to 2 servings healthy fats

▸ *Clean 16 Fast day tomorrow; eat nothing after dinner tonight*

WEEK 2, DAY 2
Monday (Clean 16 Fast Day)

Breakfast

Clean 16 Fast—skip breakfast

Lunch

Chicken Tortilla Soup (page 215)

1 cup fat-free milk

1 cup fruit salad

▶ *Or your choice of any 4 servings protein, 2 servings (or more) vegetables, 2 servings fruit, 1 serving grains, and 1 serving healthy fats*

Afternoon Snack

2 stalks celery spread with 2 tablespoons peanut butter

▶ *Or your choice of any 1 serving (or more) vegetables and 1 serving nuts/seeds*

Dinner

Brazilian Feijoada (page 227) served over ½ cup brown rice or quinoa

Tossed side salad made with 2 cups spring greens, ½ cup grape tomatoes, 1 tablespoon salad dressing

▶ *Or your choice of any 4 servings protein, 2 servings (or more) vegetables, 1 serving grains, and 1 to 2 servings healthy fats*

WEEK 2, DAY 3

Tuesday (Nonfast Day)

. . . .

Breakfast

1 cup mixed berries

Any Veggie Egg Scramble (page 201) made with green veggies (spinach, broccoli, and zucchini) served over 1 slice whole wheat toast

▶ *Or your choice of any 2 servings protein, 2 servings fruit, and 1 serving grains*

Lunch

Loaded Shrimp Ceviche (page 227)

1 apple

1 ounce whole grain crackers

▶ *Or your choice of any 4 servings protein, 2 servings (or more) vegetables, 1 serving fruit, 1 serving grains, and 1 serving healthy fats*

Afternoon Snack

½ cup (or more) baby carrots

1 ounce almonds

▶ *Or your choice of any 1 serving (or more) vegetables and 1 serving nuts/seeds*

Dinner

Latin Beans and Quinoa with Poached Eggs (page 228)

Tossed side salad made with 2 cups baby spinach, sliced red onion, 1 tablespoon olive oil, and ½ tablespoon white wine vinegar

▶ *Or your choice of any 4 servings protein, 2 servings (or more) vegetables, 1 serving grains, and 1 to 2 servings healthy fats*

▶ *Clean 16 Fast day tomorrow; eat nothing after dinner tonight*

WEEK 2, DAY 4
Wednesday (Clean 16 Fast Day)

Breakfast

Clean 16 Fast—skip breakfast

Lunch

Creamy Corn-Spinach Soup (page 216)

Whole grain dinner roll

1 cup fat-free milk

1 cup berries

▶ *Or your choice of any 4 servings protein, 2 servings (or more) vegetables, 2 servings fruit, 1 serving grains, and 1 serving healthy fats*

AFTERNOON SNACK

½ cup (or more) cherry tomatoes

1 ounce peanuts

▶ *Or your choice of any 1 serving (or more) vegetables and 1 serving nuts/seeds*

Dinner

Jamaican Jerk Salmon with Orange-Cilantro Salad (page 208) and ½ cup cooked brown rice

▶ *Or your choice of any 4 servings protein, 2 servings (or more) vegetables, 1 serving grains, and 1 to 2 servings healthy fats*

WEEK 2, DAY 5

Thursday (Nonfast Day)

. . . .

Breakfast

1 ounce whole grain cold cereal with 1 cup fat-free milk and 1 cup blueberries

▶ *Or your choice of any 2 servings protein, 2 servings fruit, and 1 serving grains*

Lunch

Latin Chicken Salad (page 205)

1 small orange

1 ounce whole grain crackers

▶ *Or your choice of any 4 servings protein, 2 servings (or more) vegetables, 1 serving fruit, 1 serving grains, and 1 serving healthy fats*

Afternoon Snack

½ cup (or more) sliced cucumbers

1 ounce chopped almonds

▶ *Or your choice of any 1 serving (or more) vegetables and 1 serving nuts/seeds*

Dinner

Arroz con Pollo (page 229)

1 cup asparagus sautéed in ½ tablespoon olive oil

▶ *Or your choice of any 4 servings protein, 2 servings (or more) vegetables, 1 serving grains, and 1 to 2 servings healthy fats*

▶ *Clean 16 Fast day tomorrow; eat nothing after dinner tonight*

WEEK 2, DAY 6
Friday (Clean 16 Fast Day and Mojito Day)

Breakfast

Clean 16 Fast—skip breakfast

Lunch

Veggie Cheese Salad (page 210)

1 cup fat-free milk

1 ounce whole grain crackers

1 cup mixed berries

▶ *Or your choice of any 4 servings protein, 2 servings (or more) vegetables, 2 servings fruit, 1 serving grains, and 1 serving healthy fats*

Afternoon Snack

½ cup (or more) baby carrots

1 ounce walnuts

▶ *Or your choice of any 1 serving (or more) vegetables and 1 serving nuts/seeds*

Dinner

Pork Fajitas with Salsa Crema (page 230)

½ small baked sweet potato

▶ *Or your choice of any 4 servings protein, 2 servings (or more) vegetables, 1 serving grains, and 1 to 2 servings healthy fats*

WEEK 2, DAY 7

Saturday (Nonfast Day and Mojito Day)

. . . .

Breakfast

1 cup melon cubes

Any Veggie Egg Scramble (page 201) made with pico de gallo veggies (tomatoes, red onions, bell peppers, and cilantro)

1 slice whole grain toast

▶ *Or your choice of any 2 servings protein, 2 servings fruit, and 1 serving grains*

Lunch

Callaloo Soup with Plantain and Crab (page 216)

1 whole grain dinner roll

1 small banana

▶ *Or your choice of any 4 servings protein, 2 servings (or more) vegetables, 1 serving fruit, 1 serving grains, and 1 serving healthy fats*

Afternoon Snack

2 large celery stalks spread with 2 tablespoons almond butter

▶ *Or your choice of any 1 serving (or more) vegetables and 1 serving nuts/seeds*

Dinner

Latin Stuffed Peppers (page 231)

▶ *Or your choice of any 4 servings protein, 2 servings (or more) vegetables, 1 serving grains, and 1 to 2 servings healthy fats*

Reward: 1 mojito! OR 1 other alcoholic beverage OR 1 serving dessert

Design Your Own Clean 16 Fast Plan

As in Week 1, if you prefer to plan your own meals, you can feel free to do so. To create your own plan, use the following weekly serving guidelines and the Mojito Diet Food Charts starting on page 153. Choose what you'd like to eat for breakfast, lunch, dinner, and snacks, remembering not to go over the recommended daily limit. Be sure you're familiar with portion sizes and the types of foods included in each food group.

As you plan your meals, remember that this week we're including three Clean 16 Fast days, during which you'll be skipping breakfast. Your goal on these days is to eat less food, not to squeeze a day's worth of food into a smaller number of meals. So, as you make your meal plans on your Clean 16 Fast days, be sure to leave out the equivalent of what you ordinarily eat at breakfast. For example, if you typically would have two servings of protein, one serving of grains, and one serving of fruit at breakfast, leave those out of your daily tally. And don't forget to measure your portions, to ensure that you don't eat too much or too little.

Here are your serving guidelines for this week:

FOOD GROUP	DAILY SERVINGS ON CLEAN 16 FAST DAYS	DAILY SERVINGS ON NONFASTING DAYS
Protein (lean meats, poultry, seafood, eggs, soy, dairy, beans/peas/lentils)	6 to 8*	8 to 10*
Vegetables	5 or more	5 or more
Fruit	2	3
Grains	2	3
Nuts/Seeds	1	1
Healthy Fats	2 to 3*	2 to 3*
Mojitos!	2 per week	2 per week

*Eat fewer servings for faster weight loss.

Here is a sample of just one way you could choose to plan a day of Week 2 meals:

WEEK 2 CUSTOM MEAL PLAN SAMPLE

BREAKFAST	LUNCH
Protein: 2 servings	Protein: 4 servings
Fruit: 1 serving	Vegetables: 2 or more servings
Grains: 1 serving	Fruit: 1 serving
[Omit on Clean 16 Fast days]	Grains: 1 serving
	Healthy fats: 1 serving

AFTERNOON SNACK	DINNER
Nuts/seeds: 1 serving	Protein: 4 servings
Vegetables: 1 or more servings	Vegetables: 2 or more servings
	Fruit: 1 serving
	Grains: 1 serving
	Healthy fats: 1 to 2 servings

ON MOJITO DAYS (FRIDAY AND SATURDAY): 1 mojito! OR 1 mixed drink OR 1 serving of beer or wine OR 1 serving of dessert

What's next?

After you complete the Clean 16 Fast week, you have two choices:

- If you have more weight to lose, cycle back through Grain Drop and the Clean 16 Fast, alternating weeks until you meet your weight-loss goal.

- If you've met your weight-loss goal, you can move on to the Mojito Maintenance Plan.

Keep It Off: The Mojito Maintenance Plan

If you have met your weight-loss goal, congratulations! I am so thrilled for you! You have worked hard and made so many terrific choices. You have lost your excess weight, burned off belly fat, improved your health, and lowered your risk of a long list of chronic illnesses, including heart disease. I cannot tell you how happy I am for you.

Now that you have met your weight-loss goal, you are ready to move on to my Mojito Maintenance Plan. You'll use this plan to maintain your weight loss and continue to reinforce all the great eating habits you learned during the Week 1 Grain Drop and the Week 2 Clean 16 Fast. This is a plan you can follow for the rest of your life.

The Mojito Maintenance Plan is simple: You'll follow the healthy eating plan that you ate on nonfasting days during the Week 2 Clean 16 Fast plan. Then you'll do one day of Grain Drop and one day of the Clean 16 Fast each week. That's it.

Plus, you'll reward yourself with *three* mojitos (or other drinks or desserts) per week.

As you maintain your weight loss, I suggest you get on the scale once a week. If you gain a pound or two, you can stop that weight loss in its tracks by adding an extra day or two of Grain Drop until you get back down to your goal. And if you splurge for a day, keep yourself on track by doing an extra Grain Drop day or a Clean 16 Fast the next day.

Along the way, continue to do your daily bursts of salsa dancing and other exercise (as we discussed in chapter 4), challenge any negative automatic thoughts about your body or your weight that may start popping up (chapter 2), and reward yourself for the efforts you're making to maintain your weight loss and your health (chapter 3). If at any point you find yourself slipping in any of those areas, go back and inspire yourself anew by rereading those chapters.

Highlights of the Mojito Maintenance Plan

- Eat a healthy baseline diet five days a week.

- Follow Grain Drop one day a week.

- Follow the Clean 16 Fast and skip breakfast one day a week.

- Weigh yourself once a week, and add extra Grain Drop days if you start to regain lost weight.

- Reward yourself with three mojitos!

Mojito Maintenance Plan Guidelines

Food groups and daily servings

You've become accustomed to eating foods from various categories of foods, including lean protein, vegetables, fruit, grains, nuts/seeds, and healthy fats. Continue to do this during Mojito Maintenance. Be sure to eat protein and either fruit or vegetables at every meal and snack.

Each day, you'll be aiming to eat a healthy number of servings. Although you don't have to be quite as careful with measuring and counting servings as you were while following Week 1 and Week 2 of the plan, I do suggest that you keep your daily serving counts in mind to prevent weight gain. Remember, it's easier to maintain weight loss than it is to lose weight again. Stay on top of what you eat and you'll stay at your goal weight.

As you follow the Mojito Maintenance Plan, aim for the following daily serving counts from each food group as your overall baseline:

MOJITO MAINTENANCE DAILY SERVING COUNTS

FOOD GROUP	DAILY SERVINGS (BASELINE)
Protein (lean meats, poultry, seafood, eggs, soy, dairy, beans/peas/lentils)	8 to 10*
Vegetables	5 or more
Fruit	3
Grains	3
Nuts/Seeds	1
Healthy Fats	2 to 3*
Mojitos!	3 per week

*Eat fewer servings for better weight control.

Portion sizes

You've probably become good at estimating healthy portion sizes. Keep doing that as you maintain your weight loss, but don't become complacent—it's very easy to start making mistakes when estimating portion sizes, and before you know it, you may be eating portions that are much larger than they should be. To check yourself, occasionally measure your portion sizes to be sure you're estimating accurately.

Meal plans

You can go back and use daily meal plans from Week 1 and Week 2, or you can design your own. Remember to have lean protein and fiber from vegetables or fruit at every meal and snack, and include heart-healthy foods with potassium, calcium, and magnesium in your eating plan each day. (See chapter 9 for a review of which foods are your best sources of these important blood pressure–lowering minerals.) And keep enjoying all those delicious, protein-packed, Latin-inspired recipes in the Recipe Guide.

Weigh in

I suggest that you weigh yourself once a week, on Sunday mornings. If you've stayed at your goal weight, congratulate yourself, and keep doing what you're doing. However, if your weight has gone up a pound or two, make some immediate course corrections. A good rule of thumb is to add an extra day of Grain Drop for every pound you've gained. Do this, and by next Sunday you should be back at your goal weight. If you're not, do Grain Drop for a full week.

Keep moving

Daily activity plays a very important role in weight-loss maintenance. It burns off fat and calories and makes you feel great about yourself. If you've done well with exercise so far, keep doing what you're doing. To prevent yourself from getting bored, mix things up a bit, trying new activities, switching up the tunes you dance to, signing up for a new class, and challenging yourself to get even better at whatever fitness activities you do. If you haven't been exercising, take your achievement in weight loss as a new beginning, a time to start adding activity into your life. I promise you that even if you've never exercised before, you will find a sense of satisfaction with even small amounts of activity.

Reward yourself!

During Mojito Maintenance, reward your efforts with up to three celebratory mojitos, alcoholic beverages, or desserts each week. Remember, a serving of dessert is one small slice of cake, one or two cookies, one small serving of flan, or other sweets or treats not exceeding 200 calories. And a serving of alcohol is 12 ounces of beer, 5 ounces of wine, or a drink made with a 1.5-ounce shot of distilled spirits such as rum, gin, whiskey, or vodka. When having mixed drinks, choose lower-calorie mixers such as seltzer, stevia, and 100 percent fruit juices.

Don't go back

You may be tempted, now that you've achieved your weight-loss goal, to go back to your pre–Mojito Diet style of eating. I urge you not to do this, because you'll very likely gain back all your lost weight—and perhaps more. You can splurge once in a while, but if you do, follow up your splurge day with a day or two on the Grain Drop plan.

Now you know everything you need to do to maintain your weight loss for life. You should be very proud of yourself for the steps you've taken to improve your health. Stay committed to your journey, and continue to celebrate and enjoy every minute of your life!

PART FOUR

THE MOJITO DIET RECIPE GUIDE

Welcome to the Mojito Diet Recipe Guide.

In the following pages, you'll find many delicious Latin-inspired recipes that fit perfectly into the Mojito Diet. These recipes combine the healthy foods I recommend throughout this book with spices, flavors, and cooking traditions from Puerto Rico, Mexico, Cuba, Brazil, Spain, Jamaica, and South America. You'll be amazed at how delicious healthy food can taste.

And, of course, you'll also find recipes for ten different kinds of mojitos, from the classic to the unconventional. You'll have to try them all!

In most cases, breakfast recipes are designed to make one serving, and main course recipes will serve four. Each recipe is followed by a tally of the number of servings from each Mojito Diet food group.

Feel free to use the Mojito Diet Food Charts beginning on page 153 to make substitutions to suit your preferences. Go ahead and swap shrimp for chicken, kidney beans for black beans, baby kale for spinach, or Gouda for cheddar cheese. And add more spice if it's what you like! Just be sure to keep an eye on portion sizes so you don't slow down your weight loss.

Mojitos

Simple Stevia Syrup 190
Simple Sugar Syrup 191
Dr. Juan's Classic Mojito 192
Very Berry Mojito 192
Mango-Pineapple Mojito 193
Blood Orange Citrus
    Mojito 194

Double Melon Mojito 194
Basil-Blackberry Mojito 195
Cucumber-Basil Mojito 196
Grapefruit Tequila Mojito 196
Chocolate Mojito 197
Pumpkin Spice Mojito 198
Mojito Water 198

Breakfast

Any Fruit Parfait 200
Any Veggie Egg Scramble 201
Any Fruit Smoothie 202
Dr. Juan's "Hulk" Protein
    Shake 202

Any Fruit Salad with
    Fresh Cheese 203
Family Breakfast Bake 203
Sweet Potato Avocado
    Toast with Egg 204

Salads

Latin Chicken Salad 205
Spanish Veggie Salad with
    Tuna and Potatoes 206
Hearty Tomato Salad with
    Black Beans 207
Cactus Paddle Salad 207
Jamaican Jerk Salmon with
    Orange-Cilantro Salad 208

The Whatever Salad
    Bowl 209
Veggie Cheese Salad 210
Papaya–Black Bean
    Chicken Salad 210
Dr. Juan's Salsa 211
Hearts of Palm with
    Crab Salad 212

Soups

Gazpacho with Pinto Beans
    and Avocado 212
Mexican Black Bean
    Soup 213

Caribbean Pumpkin Soup
    with Chickpeas 214
Chicken Tortilla Soup 215
Creamy Corn-Spinach Soup 216

Mojitos

The mojito is a traditional Cuban cocktail that is hugely popular in Miami. A classic mojito recipe pairs mint, rum, and fresh lime juice with simple syrup (made with either sugar or stevia), seltzer, and ice. But there are countless other ways to make a mojito. You can swap in other herbs instead of mint, use different fruits or even vegetables in addition to or instead of lime, and add extra flavor with spices or extracts.

As for the rum, you can go with light rum, dark rum, or any kind of flavored rum. You don't even have to use rum—feel free to substitute tequila, vodka, or other types of liquor. Use your imagination or try my recipes.

It's easiest to make mojitos with a muddler, which is a bar tool that is used to press the flavorful oils out of mint leaves and other ingredients. You can buy inexpensive muddlers in kitchen or bar supply stores. If you don't have a muddler, you can use a pestle or even the end of a wooden spoon. After muddling, you can strain out the crushed mint if you like, but most Miamians and other mojito aficionados leave it in the drink.

Mojitos are usually made with simple syrup, a sweetener made either with sugar and water or stevia and water. You can buy simple syrup or easily make your own using the recipes that follow.

Simple Stevia Syrup *Makes about 1½ cups*

Using stevia, which is a natural sweetener that is many times sweeter than sugar, saves about 64 calories when used in a mojito instead of sugar. Although stevia doesn't taste exactly the same as sugar, many people find they like it just as well, or can get used to it fairly easily. You may have to experiment with the amount of stevia you use to make simple syrup, because the sweet taste can vary by brand. You can also buy ready-made stevia syrup at some grocery stores or liquor retailers.

3 tablespoons stevia (or more or less to taste)

1½ cups boiling water

Spoon the stevia into a heatproof jar or cup. Pour the water into the jar and stir.

Allow the syrup to cool, stirring occasionally. Stevia should dissolve fairly quickly.

Cover and store in refrigerator for up to 4 weeks.

Simple Sugar Syrup *Makes about 1½ cups*

Although you can make a mojito with sugar right out of the sugar bowl, you'll have to allow a few minutes for the sugar to dissolve—otherwise you risk ending up with a crunchy mojito. It's better to make up a batch of simple syrup and keep it in the refrigerator for future use. You can also buy ready-made simple syrup in a bottle, but it's cheaper to make it yourself.

1 cup water

1 cup sugar

Combine the water and sugar in a small saucepan.

Bring to a boil. Reduce the heat and simmer, stirring often, until the sugar dissolves, 2 to 3 minutes.

Let cool, then pour into a jar. Cover and store in the refrigerator for up to 4 weeks.

> **QUICK-FIX SIMPLE SYRUP:** No simple syrup on hand? No problem. To make quick Simple Stevia Syrup, combine about ¾ teaspoon stevia and 2 tablespoons water and stir until dissolved. Use more or less stevia to taste. To make quick Simple Sugar Syrup, combine 4 teaspoons sugar and 2 tablespoons water and stir until dissolved.

Dr. Juan's Classic Mojito *Serves 1*

Enjoy the classic mojito as is or use it as a starting point to make your own custom mojito.

6 to 10 fresh mint leaves, plus 1 sprig for garnish

1 small lime, halved, plus a wedge for garnish

2 tablespoons Simple Stevia Syrup (page 190) or Simple Sugar Syrup (page 191)

1 shot (1 ½ ounces) white rum

1 cup ice

½ cup seltzer water

Place the mint leaves in a sturdy glass. Squeeze in the juice from both halves of the lime. Use a muddler to gently crush the mint well and release its flavorful oils.

Stir in the simple syrup and rum. Strain if desired.

Add the ice and seltzer water. Stir.

Garnish the glass with a mint sprig and lime wedge.

Very Berry Mojito *Serves 1*

Use whichever berries you have on hand for this summery mojito. After muddling them with the mint, leave them in the glass or strain them out. If the berries are frozen, pop them in the microwave for a few seconds to soften them before using.

6 to 10 fresh mint leaves, plus 1 sprig for garnish

1 small lime, halved, plus a wedge for garnish

¼ cup berries (any combination of blueberries, raspberries, strawberries, blackberries), plus a few extra berries for garnish

2 tablespoons Simple Stevia Syrup (page 190) or Simple Sugar Syrup (page 191)

1 shot (1 ½ ounces) white rum

1 cup ice

½ cup seltzer water

Place the mint leaves in a sturdy glass. Squeeze in the juice from both halves of the lime. Use a muddler to gently crush the mint well and release its flavorful oils.

Add the berries and gently crush with the muddler until the berries release their juices.

Stir in the simple syrup and rum. Strain if desired (although I like to leave the berries and mint in the glass).

Add the ice and seltzer water. Stir.

Garnish the glass with a mint sprig and lime wedge, and float berries on top of the drink.

Mango-Pineapple Mojito *Serves 1*

Pineapple-flavored rum adds an extra boost of flavor to this mojito, but if you don't have it, go ahead and use white rum instead. Use pineapple mint if you can find it at your local garden center. Be sure to use ripe mango—frozen is fine, just soften it in the microwave first.

6 to 10 fresh mint leaves, plus 1 sprig for garnish

1 small lime, halved, plus a wedge for garnish

¼ cup chopped ripe mango, plus a few extra small chunks for garnish

2 tablespoons pineapple juice

2 tablespoons Simple Stevia Syrup (page 190) or Simple Sugar Syrup (page 191)

1 shot (1½ ounces) pineapple-flavored rum or white rum

1 cup ice

⅓ cup seltzer water

Place the mint leaves in a sturdy glass. Squeeze in the juice from both halves of the lime. Use a muddler to gently crush the mint well and release its flavorful oils.

Add the mango and gently crush with the muddler.

Stir in the pineapple juice, simple syrup, and rum. Strain if desired (although I like to leave the mango and mint in the glass).

Add the ice and seltzer water. Stir.

Garnish the glass with a mint sprig and lime wedge, and float mango chunks on top of the drink.

Blood Orange Citrus Mojito *Serves 1*

Blood orange gives this mojito a lovely reddish color. The blood orange's unique ruby-colored flesh is due to the presence of anthocyanins, compounds that are believed to have health-supporting benefits.

- 6 to 10 fresh mint leaves, plus 1 sprig for garnish
- 1 small lime, halved
- ½ small lemon
- Juice of 1 small blood orange (about ¼ cup), plus a slice for garnish
- 2 tablespoons Simple Stevia Syrup (page 190) or Simple Sugar Syrup (page 191)
- 1 shot (1 ½ ounces) white rum
- 1 cup ice
- ⅓ cup seltzer water

Place the mint leaves in a sturdy glass. Squeeze in the juice from the lime halves and lemon. Use a muddler to gently crush the mint well and release its flavorful oils.

Stir in the blood orange juice, simple syrup, and rum. Strain if desired. Add the ice and seltzer water. Stir.

Garnish the glass with a mint sprig and blood orange slice.

Double Melon Mojito *Serves 1*

Use whichever melon you have on hand for this refreshing mojito. You can also opt to use melon-flavored rum.

- 6 to 10 fresh mint leaves, plus 1 sprig for garnish
- 1 small lime, halved, plus a wedge for garnish
- ¼ cup chopped melon (use two types, such as cantaloupe, honeydew, or watermelon), plus a few extra small chunks for garnish
- 2 tablespoons Simple Stevia Syrup (page 190) or Simple Sugar Syrup (page 191)
- 1 shot (1 ½ ounces) white rum or melon-flavored rum
- 1 cup ice
- ½ cup seltzer water

Place the mint leaves in a sturdy glass. Squeeze in the juice from both halves of the lime. Use a muddler to gently crush the mint well and release its flavorful oils.

Add the melon and gently crush with the muddler.

Stir in the simple syrup and rum. Strain if desired.

Add the ice and seltzer water. Stir.

Garnish the glass with a mint sprig and lime wedge, and float the small melon chunks on top of the drink.

Basil-Blackberry Mojito *Serves 1*

This recipe replaces mint with basil for a delicious, unique taste. It's also wonderful made with fresh strawberries.

6 to 10 fresh basil leaves, plus 1 sprig for garnish

1 small lime, halved, plus a wedge for garnish

¼ cup blackberries, plus a few extra berries for garnish

2 tablespoons Simple Stevia Syrup (page 190) or Simple Sugar Syrup (page 191)

1 shot (1½ ounces) white rum

1 cup ice

½ cup seltzer water

Place the basil leaves in a sturdy glass. Squeeze in the juice from both halves of the lime. Use a muddler to gently crush the basil well and release its flavorful oils.

Add the blackberries and gently crush with the muddler until the berries release their juices.

Stir in the simple syrup and rum. Strain if desired.

Add the ice and seltzer water. Stir.

Garnish the glass with a basil sprig and lime wedge, and float berries on top of the drink.

Cucumber-Basil Mojito *Serves 1*

Cucumbers and basil combine to create an exhilarating flavor in this mojito. This drink is delicious served with gazpacho or any kind of salad.

6 to 10 fresh basil leaves, plus 1 sprig for garnish

1 small lime, halved, plus a wedge for garnish

¼ cup finely chopped peeled and seeded cucumber, plus 1 slice for garnish

2 tablespoons Simple Stevia Syrup (page 190) or Simple Sugar Syrup (page 191)

1 shot (1½ ounces) white rum

1 cup ice

½ cup seltzer water

Place the basil leaves in a sturdy glass. Squeeze in the juice from both halves of the lime. Use a muddler to gently crush the basil well and release its flavorful oils.

Add the cucumber and crush well with the muddler.

Stir in the simple syrup and rum. Strain if desired.

Add the ice and seltzer water. Stir.

Garnish the glass with a basil sprig and cucumber slice.

Grapefruit Tequila Mojito *Serves 1*

Who says you have to use rum in a mojito? Swap tequila for rum, and add a splash of grapefruit for a delicious twist.

6 to 10 fresh mint leaves, plus 1 sprig for garnish

1 small lime, halved, plus a wedge for garnish

2 tablespoons grapefruit juice

2 tablespoons Simple Stevia Syrup (page 190) or Simple Sugar Syrup (page 191)

1 shot (1½ ounces) tequila

1 cup ice

⅓ cup seltzer water

Place the mint leaves in a sturdy glass. Squeeze in the juice from both halves of the lime. Use a muddler to gently crush the mint well and release its flavorful oils.

Stir in the grapefruit juice, simple syrup, and tequila. Strain if desired.

Add the ice and seltzer water. Stir.

Garnish the glass with a mint sprig and lime wedge.

Chocolate Mojito *Serves 1*

This recipe calls for chocolate mint, which is available at some grocery stores. If you like to grow your own herbs, look for chocolate mint plants at nurseries or garden centers. The recipe also calls for pure chocolate extract, which is available at some grocery stores and gourmet food shops. To make the chocolate shavings, use a cheese grater or vegetable peeler to shave a touch of dark chocolate over the drink.

6 to 10 fresh chocolate mint leaves, plus 1 sprig for garnish

1 small lime, halved, plus a wedge for garnish

2 tablespoons Simple Stevia Syrup (page 190) or Simple Sugar Syrup (page 191)

1 shot (1½ ounces) white rum

2 to 3 drops pure chocolate extract

1 cup ice

½ cup seltzer water

Dark chocolate shavings, for garnish (optional)

Place the chocolate mint leaves in a sturdy glass. Squeeze in the juice from both halves of the lime. Use a muddler to gently crush the mint well and release its flavorful oils.

Stir in the simple syrup, rum, and chocolate extract. Strain if desired. Add the ice and seltzer water. Stir.

Garnish the glass with a chocolate mint sprig, lime wedge, and chocolate shavings (if using).

Pumpkin Spice Mojito *Serves 1*

This definitely isn't your typical Miami mojito. But it's a nice change of pace, especially in the fall when temperatures start to drop. Dark rum and orange juice complement the autumnal flavors of the pumpkin and cinnamon.

6 to 10 fresh mint leaves, plus 1 sprig for garnish

2 tablespoons orange juice

1 tablespoon light brown sugar

1 tablespoon canned unsweetened pumpkin puree

Dash of cinnamon (or use pumpkin pie spice or allspice)

1 shot (1 ½ ounces) dark rum

1 cup ice

⅓ cup seltzer water

Orange slice, for garnish (optional)

Place the mint leaves in a sturdy glass. Add the orange juice and brown sugar. Use a muddler to gently crush the mint well and release its flavorful oils. Let the mixture sit for a few minutes, mixing occasionally until the brown sugar dissolves.

Stir in the pumpkin puree and cinnamon.

Add the rum and mix well.

Add the ice and seltzer water. Stir.

Garnish the glass with a mint sprig and orange slice (if using).

Mojito Water *Makes 4 cups*

Mojito Water is an excellent beverage for fasting, for drinking throughout the day, or as an alternative for people who love the taste of lime and mint but choose not to drink alcohol.

20 fresh mint leaves, or 4 mint tea bags (if you don't have fresh mint)

1 cup boiling water

Juice of 2 limes

3 cups cold water

Bruise the mint leaves by bunching them up with your fingers to break them apart slightly, allowing them to release their oils.

In a heat-safe 1 ½–quart pitcher, combine the boiling water and mint leaves or tea bags. Allow to steep for 10 minutes.

If you're using fresh mint, leave it in the pitcher, but if you're using tea bags, remove them.

Stir in the lime juice and cold water. Refrigerate until ready to drink.

DR. JUAN'S WISDOM

GROW YOUR OWN

Mint is easy to grow on a sunny windowsill or in a patio container or garden. Although spearmint is the type of mint most commonly used in mojitos—in fact, spearmint is sometimes labeled "mojito mint" in garden centers—many other kinds of mint are available, including peppermint, chocolate mint, pineapple mint, apple mint, orange mint, lemon mint, ginger mint, and even licorice mint.

You can grow mint from seeds or buy seedlings from a nursery. You can also start new mint plants by taking a cutting from an existing plant, setting it in water for a few weeks until it roots, and then planting it in soil.

Mint is a vigorous perennial that will reappear each spring in most planting zones. It is happiest growing in soil that is kept moist, and although it does tolerate some shade, it also needs sun. If you grow mint outdoors, be sure to prune it often to prevent it from overtaking your garden.

In addition to mojitos, fresh mint can be used in salads, pesto, fresh vegetable dishes, fruit salad, and sauces served with lamb or fish.

Breakfast

Any Fruit Parfait *Serves 1*

▶ (GRAIN DROP and CLEAN 16)

Parfaits are a delicious way to start the day. By combining yogurt with fruit and nuts, you fill up on protein and fiber, and also get calcium, potassium, and other important nutrients. For a more filling breakfast—and even more fiber—add nuts or, on days when you're eating grains, whole grain granola. Sprinkle in spices for an unexpected burst of flavor.

1 single-serve container plain fat-free yogurt

Dash of spice (cinnamon, ginger, nutmeg, allspice, apple pie spice, or pumpkin pie spice)

1 cup chopped soft fruit, such as berries, cherries, banana, papaya, pineapple, peach, mango, etc.

1 ounce chopped nuts, such as walnuts, almonds, pecans, or macadamia nuts (optional, on Grain Drop days) OR ¼ cup whole grain granola (optional)

Mix the yogurt and spice.

Spoon half of the yogurt into a parfait glass or bowl. Top with half of the fruit. If using, top with half of the nuts or granola. Repeat using the remaining yogurt, fruit, and nuts or granola.

PER SERVING: Protein: 1, Fruit: 2, Grains: 1 (if using granola), Nuts: 1 (if using nuts)

Any Veggie Egg Scramble *Serves 1*

▶ (GRAIN DROP and CLEAN 16)

Eggs are an excellent source of protein and a quick, easy way to get going in the morning. Add vegetables, herbs, and spices and you'll turn simple scrambled eggs into a tasty breakfast that also delivers fiber and a mix of vitamins and minerals.

2 eggs

1 tablespoon chopped fresh herbs, such as cilantro, oregano, or basil (or a sprinkle of dried herbs)

Cooking spray

1 cup (or more) chopped fresh vegetables, such as onions, red bell peppers, green bell peppers, tomatoes, spinach, broccoli, mushrooms, zucchini, green chilies, etc.

Dash of spice, such as chili powder, ground cumin, red pepper flakes, cayenne pepper, etc. (optional)

¼ cup shredded cheese (optional)

Whisk together the eggs and herbs in a small bowl until frothy.

Coat a small skillet with cooking spray and set the skillet over medium heat. Add the vegetables and sauté for a few minutes or until tender. Sprinkle with spices, if using.

Pour the egg mixture over the vegetables and cook, stirring gently, to desired doneness. If using cheese, reduce the heat, sprinkle the cheese over the eggs, and heat for 1 minute to allow the cheese to melt.

PER SERVING: Protein: 2 (3 if using cheese), Vegetables: 2

Any Fruit Smoothie *Serves 1*

▶ (GRAIN DROP and CLEAN 16)

Fruit smoothies are the ultimate healthy fast-food breakfast. Toss a few ingredients in the blender, give it a whir, pour it into a travel cup, and you're good to go. Or whip it up the night before and refrigerate overnight. To make it even healthier, toss in some baby greens. And to give it an extra protein boost, add nut butter, such as peanut or almond butter.

- 1 single-serve container plain fat-free yogurt,* Greek or regular
- 1 cup cut-up fruit, fresh or frozen, preferably softer fruits such as banana, mango, berries, papaya, pineapple, peach, etc.
- 1 cup baby spinach or baby kale (optional)
- 2 tablespoons nut butter (optional)
- Ice (optional)

Place all the ingredients in a blender or smoothie maker. Blend until smooth.

If needed, add water to reach the desired consistency.

Alternatively: Use 1 cup fat-free milk, 1 cup soy milk, 1 cup almond milk, or 1 cup kefir (a fermented milk drink)

PER SERVING: Protein: 1, Vegetables: 1 (if using spinach or kale), Fruit: 2, Nuts/seeds: 1 (if using nut butter)

Dr. Juan's "Hulk" Protein Shake *Serves 1*

▶ (GRAIN DROP and CLEAN 16)

This is my favorite protein shake—I love drinking it after working out. The combination of peanut butter and protein powder gives me loads of energy and keeps me feeling full for hours.

- 1 medium banana, peeled and frozen
- 1 cup almond milk
- 2 teaspoons peanut butter
- 1 scoop protein powder

Combine all the ingredients in a blender and blend until smooth.

PER SERVING: Protein: 4, Fruit: 2, Nuts: 1

Any Fruit Salad with Fresh Cheese *Serves 1*

▶ (GRAIN DROP and CLEAN 16)

Fruit combines perfectly with fresh cheeses to make a breakfast that contains healthy amounts of protein, calcium, fiber, vitamins, and minerals. To add even more flavor, sprinkle with fresh herbs or a dash of spice.

1 cup chopped fruit, such as apples, oranges, pears, peaches, berries, bananas, mangoes, papayas, etc.

Dash of spice, such as cinnamon, nutmeg, ginger, allspice, chili powder, etc. (optional)

½ cup low-fat fresh cheese, such as such as cottage cheese, Queso Fresco, cotija, Panela, or ricotta

1 tablespoon chopped fresh herbs, such as mint, basil, or oregano (optional)

Mix the fruit with the spice (if using).

Scoop the cheese into a bowl and top with the fruit and fresh herbs (if using).

PER SERVING: Protein: 1, Fruit: 2

Family Breakfast Bake *Serves 4*

▶ (GRAIN DROP and CLEAN 16)

This recipe bakes up a protein- and veggie-rich weekend breakfast that's good for the whole family. Or bake it in the evening, cut it into single servings, and refrigerate for 4 days of quick weekday breakfasts. To reheat, warm it up in the microwave for 30 seconds to 1 minute on medium power.

Cooking spray

4 cups (about 4 ounces) baby spinach

¼ cup chopped red onion

½ cup chopped yellow bell pepper

½ cup chopped red bell pepper

1 cup chopped tomato or halved grape tomatoes

6 eggs, whisked well

½ cup fat-free milk

½ cup shredded cheddar or Pepper Jack cheese

1 teaspoon chili powder

Freshly ground black pepper

(continued)

Coat a 1-quart baking dish with cooking spray.

Preheat the oven to 350°F.

Coat a large skillet with cooking spray. Set over medium heat, add the spinach, and sauté for a few minutes, stirring often, just until the spinach is wilted. Drain well in a colander. Leave the spinach in the colander to cool slightly.

Coat the skillet with cooking spray again. Add the onion and bell peppers and sauté for a few minutes over medium heat, stirring often, just until the vegetables are tender.

Transfer the spinach and sautéed vegetables to a bowl. Add the tomatoes, eggs, milk, cheese, chili powder, and pepper to taste. Mix well and pour into the baking dish.

Bake for about 50 minutes, or until a knife inserted in the center comes out clean.

PER SERVING: Protein: 2, Vegetables: 2

Sweet Potato Avocado Toast with Egg *Serves 1*

▶ (GRAIN DROP and CLEAN 16)

Sweet potatoes are one of the most nutritious foods you can eat, packed with beta-carotene, potassium, and fiber. In this recipe, they take over for toast and are deliciously topped with guacamole, which is another nutrient-rich superstar. This is a breakfast that will keep you going all morning.

1 narrow sweet potato, 5 inches long, unpeeled

Cooking spray

2 eggs

¼ cup guacamole

Freshly ground black pepper

Halve the sweet potato lengthwise (save one half for another use). Cut the sweet potato half lengthwise into ¼-inch-thick slices.

Place the sweet potato slices in the toaster and toast on the highest setting until the slices are tender. (This may require several rounds of toasting, up to about 5 minutes total.) Allow the sweet potato slices to cool slightly.

(continued)

Coat a small skillet with cooking spray. Set over medium heat and cook the eggs over easy.

Spread the sweet potato slices with the guacamole. Top with the eggs and a sprinkling of pepper.

PER SERVING: Protein: 2, Vegetables: 1, Healthy fats: 1

Salads

Latin Chicken Salad *Serves 4*

▶ (GRAIN DROP and CLEAN 16)

Steaming the chicken makes it supremely tender in this veggie-rich salad.

1 ¼ pounds boneless, skinless chicken breasts

1 pound new potatoes, unpeeled, diced

¼ pound green beans, trimmed and cut into 1-inch pieces

2 cups chopped mixed fresh vegetables (your choice of carrots, celery, snow peas, bell peppers, broccoli, corn, mushrooms, tomatoes, or whatever else you would enjoy)

4 dill pickle spears, diced

1 medium avocado, pitted and peeled

1 cup fat-free buttermilk

¼ cup chopped fresh cilantro

1 tablespoon fresh lemon juice

4 cups baby salad greens

Place the chicken in a steamer basket over a pot of boiling water. Cover and steam for 8 to 10 minutes or until just cooked through. Transfer the chicken to a plate to cool.

Arrange the potatoes in the same steamer basket. Cover and steam for 8 minutes. Add the beans and steam for 5 minutes longer. Transfer the potatoes and beans to a large bowl to cool.

Tear the chicken into small pieces and add to the potato mixture. Add the fresh vegetables and pickles.

(continued)

Place the avocado, buttermilk, cilantro, and lemon juice in a blender. Blend until smooth. Add the dressing to the chicken salad and toss to coat.

To serve, divide the salad greens among 4 plates. Spoon an even portion of chicken salad on top.

PER SERVING: Protein: 4, Vegetables: 3, Healthy fats: 1

Spanish Veggie Salad with Tuna and Potatoes *Serves 4*

▶ (GRAIN DROP and CLEAN 16)

Refreshing yet filling, this salad makes a terrific lunch or light dinner.

½ pound small red potatoes, scrubbed

4 eggs

1 medium head romaine lettuce, cut crosswise into thin ribbons

4 plum tomatoes, quartered

1 medium cucumber, sliced

1 red bell pepper, cut into thin strips

1 (15-ounce) can water-packed artichoke hearts, drained, each quartered

2 (5-ounce) cans water-packed chunk light tuna, drained

20 small pitted green olives, sliced

2 teaspoons mustard

1 tablespoon red wine vinegar

3 tablespoons olive oil

Place the potatoes and eggs in a medium saucepan with water to cover. Bring to a boil, reduce the heat to medium, and cook for 10 minutes, or until a sharp knife easily slides through a potato.

Drain the eggs and potatoes. Peel the eggs and let cool. When the potatoes and eggs are cool enough to handle, quarter them.

Lay out 4 plates and arrange an even portion of lettuce on each plate, followed by an even portion of potato and egg wedges, tomatoes, cucumbers, bell peppers, artichoke hearts, tuna, and olives.

Whisk together the mustard and vinegar. Whisk in the oil until blended. Drizzle the dressing over each salad.

PER SERVING: Protein: 3, Vegetables: 4, Healthy fats: 1

Hearty Tomato Salad with Black Beans *Serves 4*

▶ (GRAIN DROP and CLEAN 16)

Serve this chunky salad over mixed greens for even more fiber and nutrition.

1 (15-ounce) can black beans, rinsed and drained

1 (14-ounce) can hearts of palm, drained and sliced

4 medium tomatoes, cut into chunks

1 cup thinly sliced fennel

1 green bell pepper, thinly sliced

10 large pitted black olives, sliced

1 tablespoon olive oil

2 teaspoons sherry vinegar

1 ounce Manchego cheese, grated

Place the black beans, hearts of palm, tomatoes, fennel, bell pepper, and olives in a salad bowl. Drizzle the oil and vinegar over the mixture. Add the cheese and gently toss to combine.

Spoon an even portion of salad into 4 large salad bowls.

PER SERVING: Protein: 1, Vegetables: 3, Healthy fats: ½

Cactus Paddle Salad *Serves 4*

▶ (GRAIN DROP and CLEAN 16)

Prickly pear cactus paddles taste a little like green beans—in fact, you can substitute green beans if you'd like. Some specialty markets sell fresh cactus paddles, but they're easier to find in jars or cans. Just be sure to drain and rinse them to remove excess salt. In this traditional Latin salad, these vegetables are paired with pinto beans and cheese.

1 (30-ounce) can or jar sliced cactus paddles,* rinsed and drained

1 (15-ounce) can pinto beans, rinsed and drained

1 cup halved cherry tomatoes

1 cup chopped cucumber

½ cup chopped radishes

¼ cup minced red onion

20 small or 10 large pitted Spanish olives, chopped

½ cup crumbled Queso Fresco or feta cheese

2 tablespoons fresh lime juice

2 tablespoons olive oil

(continued)

Alternatively: Use 1 pound green beans, steamed and cut into bite-size pieces

Combine all the ingredients in a large bowl. Gently toss to mix. Spoon an even portion onto 4 plates.

PER SERVING: Protein: 1, Vegetables: 3, Healthy fats: 1

Jamaican Jerk Salmon with Orange-Cilantro Salad *Serves 4*

▶ (GRAIN DROP and CLEAN 16)

Scotch bonnet peppers are extremely fiery. If you prefer milder heat, substitute a jalapeño.

FOR THE JERK SALMON:

- 3 tablespoons fresh lime juice
- 3 tablespoons olive oil
- 2 cloves garlic, minced
- 2 teaspoons grated fresh ginger
- 1 Scotch bonnet pepper, stemmed, seeded, and minced
- ½ teaspoon ground allspice
- ¼ teaspoon ground cinnamon
- ¼ teaspoon salt
- 1¼ pounds salmon, cut into 4 equal-size fillets
- Cooking spray

FOR THE SALAD:

- 8 cups chopped romaine lettuce
- 2 medium oranges, peeled, separated into segments, and cut into bite-size pieces
- ½ medium cucumber, chopped
- ¼ cup chopped fresh cilantro

To make the salmon, whisk together the lime juice, oil, garlic, ginger, Scotch bonnet, allspice, cinnamon, and salt in a bowl. Coat the salmon flesh with 1 tablespoon of the jerk sauce. Set the remaining mixture aside to dress the salad.

Coat a large nonstick skillet with cooking spray and place over medium heat. Place the salmon, skin side down, in the pan and cook for 6 minutes. Cover the pan and cook for 4 to 5 minutes more, or until the fish is just cooked through. Transfer the salmon to a plate, sliding a spatula between the fish and skin, which should have stuck to the pan. Tent the fish with foil.

(continued)

To make the salad, place the romaine in a salad bowl. Add the remaining jerk sauce, orange pieces, cucumber, and cilantro and gently toss to mix.

Divide the salad evenly among 4 plates and top each with a salmon fillet.

PER SERVING: Protein: 4, Vegetables: 2, Fruit: 1, Healthy fats: 1

The Whatever Salad Bowl *Serves 1*

▶ (GRAIN DROP and CLEAN 16)

I call this the "whatever" salad bowl because you can make it with whatever protein, vegetables, and other ingredients you have in your kitchen. And you can have it for whatever meal you'd like — it's perfect for lunch, dinner, or even breakfast, if you don't mind moving out of the usual breakfast-food lane. You can vary the amounts of each ingredient based on your serving needs for the meal — leave out the grains if it's a Grain Drop day. It is an easy way to pack protein, fiber, and loads of nutrients into an easy-to-eat bowl.

1 cup shredded greens, such as spinach, romaine, baby kale, or spring greens

1 tablespoon salad dressing

1 cup or more of chopped vegetables, such as corn, zucchini, tomatoes, cucumbers, broccoli, jicama, etc.

½ cup cooked grain, such as brown rice or quinoa (optional; omit on Grain Drop days)

2 ounces cooked lean meat or fish, such as chicken, turkey, tuna, or shrimp, or 2 hard-boiled eggs

½ cup cooked or canned beans/peas/lentils, such as white beans, black beans, chickpeas, red lentils, etc.

¼ cup shredded cheese, such as cheddar or Jack

3 tablespoons guacamole

½ cup salsa

Place the greens in a large bowl. Toss with salad dressing.

Top with the vegetables, grain (if using), meat or fish, and beans.

Sprinkle with the cheese.

Scoop the guacamole and salsa on top.

PER SERVING: Protein: 4, Vegetables: 4, Grains: 1 (if using optional grain), Healthy fats: 1

Veggie Cheese Salad *Serves 1*

▶ (GRAIN DROP and CLEAN 16)

This is an easy, tasty lunch salad that combines cheese and veggies with a refreshing dressing. If you have the ingredients on hand, you could also add minced garlic and minced shallots to the dressing.

1 tablespoon olive oil

½ tablespoon white wine vinegar

½ teaspoon fresh lemon juice

2 ounces cubed cheese, such as cheddar or Pepper Jack

2 cups chopped veggies, such as cherry tomatoes, broccoli, red bell peppers, red onion, or zucchini

½ tablespoon chopped fresh herbs, such as parsley, cilantro, dill, or mint (or more to taste)

Whisk together the oil, vinegar, and lemon juice in a small bowl. Combine the cheese, veggies, and fresh herbs in a large bowl. Pour the dressing over the salad and toss gently.

PER SERVING: Protein: 2, Vegetables: 4, Healthy fats: 1

Papaya–Black Bean Chicken Salad *Serves 4*

▶ (GRAIN DROP and CLEAN 16)

Once you steam the chicken, this dish comes together in a snap. This recipe is also good with cold boiled shrimp instead of the chicken.

2 (5-ounce) boneless, skinless chicken breasts

2 cups diced ripe papaya

1 cup diced jícama

1 (15-ounce) can black beans, rinsed and drained

1 small avocado, pitted, peeled, and diced

4 tablespoons fresh lime juice

2 tablespoons olive oil

½ teaspoon hot sauce

¼ teaspoon salt

4 cups baby spinach

Place the chicken in a steamer basket over a pot of boiling water. Cover and steam for 8 to 10 minutes or until just cooked through. Transfer the chicken to a plate to cool. Tear into bite-size pieces.

(continued)

Combine the chicken, papaya, jícama, black beans, avocado, lime juice, oil, hot sauce, and salt in a bowl. Gently toss to mix.

Divide the spinach among 4 plates and top with an even portion of chicken salad.

PER SERVING: Protein: 3, Vegetables: 1½, Fruit: 1, Healthy fats: 1

Dr. Juan's Salsa *Serves 4*

▶ (GRAIN DROP and CLEAN 16)

I love salsa because it's such an enjoyable way to add extra vegetables and fiber to almost any food, from omelets to salads to main dishes, and it's a great dip for raw veggies you can eat at snack time. Use this recipe as a starting point, adjusting the amount of peppers, garlic, and other ingredients to taste.

- 8 plum tomatoes, cored and chopped
- ½ small red onion, chopped
- ½ green bell pepper, chopped
- 1 to 2 cloves garlic, to taste, minced
- 1 jalapeño pepper, ribs and seeds removed, finely chopped, or more to taste
- ¼ cup chopped fresh cilantro, or more to taste
- Juice of 1 lime
- ½ teaspoon ground cumin

Combine all the ingredients in a medium bowl and toss together gently.

PER SERVING: Vegetables: 2

Hearts of Palm with Crab Salad *Serves 4*

▶ (GRAIN DROP and CLEAN 16)

This elegant salad is dressy enough for company. It's easy, yet impressive.

- 1 head romaine lettuce, thinly sliced crosswise
- 1 (14-ounce) can hearts of palm, drained and sliced
- 1 medium avocado, pitted, peeled, and sliced
- 4 scallions, thinly sliced
- 12 ounces cooked crabmeat
- 4 eggs, hard-boiled, peeled, and quartered
- ¼ cup fresh lemon juice
- 2 tablespoons olive oil

Divide the romaine among 4 salad plates.

Top each serving of greens with an even portion of hearts of palm, avocado slices, scallions, crabmeat, and egg quarters.

Whisk together the lemon juice and oil. Drizzle the dressing over each salad.

PER SERVING: Protein: 4, Vegetables: 2, Healthy fats: 1 ½

Soups

Gazpacho with Pinto Beans and Avocado *Serves 4*

▶ (GRAIN DROP and CLEAN 16)

Using canned tomatoes means you can enjoy this vegetable-rich Spanish soup all year long!

- 1 (28-ounce) can crushed tomatoes
- 1 cup cold water
- 1 medium cucumber, unpeeled, cut into large pieces
- 3 bell peppers (1 green, 1 yellow, and 1 red), cored, seeded, and cut into large pieces
- 1 rib celery, cut into large pieces
- 1 clove garlic, peeled
- 2 scallions, each cut into 4 pieces
- 2 tablespoons olive oil
- 2 tablespoons balsamic vinegar
- ½ teaspoon salt
- 1 (15-ounce) can pinto beans, rinsed and drained
- 1 medium avocado, pitted, peeled, and chopped

(continued)

Place the crushed tomatoes in a large bowl and stir in the water.

Place the cucumber in a food processor, pulse until coarsely chopped, and add to the tomatoes. Place the bell peppers in the food processor, pulse until coarsely chopped, and add to the bowl. Pulse the celery, garlic, and scallions until minced and add to the gazpacho.

Stir in the oil, balsamic vinegar, and salt. Stir the soup, cover, and refrigerate, preferably for several hours.

When ready to serve, ladle even portions of gazpacho into 4 bowls. Top each serving with a portion of pinto beans and avocado.

PER SERVING: Protein: 1, Vegetables: 4, Healthy fats: 1

Mexican Black Bean Soup *Serves 4*

▶ (GRAIN DROP and CLEAN 16)

Cooks in Mexico often use avocado leaf to make this soup, but fennel works just as well (and is easy to find in most grocery stores). Serve it with a wedge of lime and hot sauce, if you wish.

- 2 tablespoons olive oil
- 1 medium onion, chopped
- 1 cup chopped fennel
- 1½ teaspoons ground cumin
- ½ teaspoon salt

- 3½ cups low-salt chicken broth
- 2 (15-ounce) cans black beans, rinsed and drained
- ½ cup crumbled Queso Fresco cheese
- ¼ cup chopped fresh cilantro

Heat the oil in a large saucepan over medium heat. Add the onion, fennel, cumin, and salt and sauté for 8 minutes, until the vegetables are soft. Add the broth and black beans, scraping up any browned bits that have stuck to the bottom of the pot. Bring the soup to a boil, then reduce the heat to medium and simmer for 15 minutes.

Let cool slightly. When the soup is cool enough to handle, transfer half to a blender and blend until smooth. Return the pureed soup to the saucepan and stir to combine.

Divide the soup among 4 bowls and top each serving with 2 tablespoons Queso Fresco and 1 tablespoon cilantro.

PER SERVING: Protein: 2, Vegetables: 1, Healthy fats: ½

Caribbean Pumpkin Soup with Chickpeas *Serves 4*

▶ (GRAIN DROP and CLEAN 16)

Chickpeas add protein to this comforting orange soup topped with crunchy roasted pumpkin seeds instead of croutons.

3 tablespoons olive oil

1 medium onion, chopped

2 cups cubed sugar pumpkin or peeled butternut squash

1 cup diced sweet potato, unpeeled

1½ teaspoons curry powder

½ teaspoon ground cinnamon

1 teaspoon salt

4 cups low-salt chicken broth

2 teaspoons canned chipotle salsa (if you can't find chipotle salsa, use chipotle peppers in adobo sauce)

1 (15-ounce) can chickpeas, rinsed and drained

4 tablespoons roasted hulled pumpkin seeds

Heat the oil in a large soup pot over medium-high heat. Add the onion, pumpkin, and sweet potato and sauté for about 8 minutes or until the vegetables begin to brown. Reduce the heat to medium. Stir in the curry powder, cinnamon, and salt and cook for 5 minutes to combine the flavors. Add the broth and salsa. Bring to a boil, then reduce the heat to medium and simmer for about 40 minutes, or until the pumpkin is tender.

Let cool slightly. When the soup is cool enough to handle, transfer it in batches to a blender and puree until smooth. Return the puree to the pot and stir in the chickpeas.

Ladle the soup into 4 bowls and sprinkle each serving with 1 tablespoon pumpkin seeds.

PER SERVING: Protein: 1, Vegetables: 2, Nuts/seeds: ½, Healthy fats: 1

Chicken Tortilla Soup *Serves 4*

▶ (CLEAN 16)

This traditional soup gets its zip from fresh cilantro and lime.

4 (6-inch) corn tortillas, each halved and cut into thin strips

Cooking spray

2 tablespoons olive oil

1 medium onion, diced

1 teaspoon ground cumin

½ teaspoon salt

3 cups low-salt chicken broth

2 cups diced fresh tomatoes

¾ pound boneless, skinless chicken breast, cut into ¼-inch-thick strips

½ cup shredded Pepper Jack cheese

¼ cup chopped fresh cilantro

1 lime, cut into 4 wedges

Preheat the oven to 400°F.

Scatter the tortilla strips in an even layer on a baking sheet and coat them with cooking spray. Bake for 12 minutes or until golden.

Heat the oil in a large saucepan over medium heat. Add the onion, cumin, and salt and sauté for 5 minutes, until the onion has softened. Stir in the broth and tomatoes. Bring the soup to a boil, then reduce the heat to medium-low and simmer for 10 minutes. Add the chicken and simmer for 2 minutes more, or until the chicken is just cooked through.

Divide the soup among 4 shallow soup bowls. Divide the tortilla chips evenly among them. Top each serving with 2 tablespoons cheese and 1 tablespoon cilantro. Serve with lime wedges.

PER SERVING: Protein: 3, Vegetables: 1, Grains: 1, Healthy fats: ½

Creamy Corn-Spinach Soup *Serves 4*

▶ (GRAIN DROP and CLEAN 16)

Blitzing half of this soup in a blender gives it a creamy consistency, while still retaining some chunkiness from the onion and corn. Instead of chicken or shrimp, you can opt to use plant-based proteins such as beans or tofu.

2 tablespoons olive oil

1 medium onion, chopped

3 cups low-salt chicken broth

3 cups corn kernels, fresh (about 4 large ears) or frozen (thawed)

2 cloves garlic, minced

6 cups baby spinach

8 ounces cooked and chopped chicken or boiled shrimp

Heat the oil in a soup pot over medium heat. Add the onion and sauté for 5 minutes until golden. Add the broth, corn, and garlic. Bring the mixture to a boil, then reduce the heat to medium-low and simmer for 10 minutes. Stir in the spinach and continue cooking for about 1 minute, until the spinach has just wilted.

Let cool slightly. When the soup is cool enough to handle, transfer half to a blender and blend until creamy and smooth. Return the puree to the pot and stir to combine.

Mix in the chicken or shrimp and divide among 4 soup bowls.

PER SERVING: Protein: 2, Vegetables: 3, Healthy fats: ½

Callaloo Soup with Plantain and Crab *Serves 4*

▶ (GRAIN DROP and CLEAN 16)

Callaloo is the name for the leafy greens, also known as amaranth, typically used in this Caribbean dish. If you can't find callaloo leaves, substitute Swiss chard leaves.

2 tablespoons olive oil

6 scallions, thinly sliced

1 yellow plantain, peeled and diced

1 Scotch bonnet pepper, stemmed, seeded, and minced

1½ teaspoons dried thyme

½ teaspoon salt

4 cups low-salt chicken broth

4 cups chopped callaloo leaves or Swiss chard leaves

(continued)

3 cloves garlic, minced

1 cup frozen sliced okra (not necessary to thaw before adding)

2 (6-ounce) cans crabmeat, drained, or 8 ounces cooked fresh crabmeat

1 cup light coconut milk

Heat the oil in a soup pot over medium heat. Add the scallions, plantain, Scotch bonnet, thyme, and salt and sauté until the vegetables are soft, about 5 minutes.

Stir in the broth and scrape up any browned bits that have stuck to the bottom of the pot. Add the callaloo and garlic. Bring the soup to a boil, then reduce the heat to low and simmer, partially covered, for 15 minutes.

Stir in the okra, crab, and coconut milk. Bring to a boil, then reduce the heat to low and simmer, partially covered, for 10 minutes more to heat through. Divide among 4 large bowls.

PER SERVING: Protein: 2, Vegetables: 2, Healthy fats: 1

Chickpea-Spinach Soup *Serves 4*

▶ (GRAIN DROP and CLEAN 16)

Spinach turns this soup a gorgeous emerald green. Cotija cheese can be found in most supermarkets; use feta if you can't find it.

2 tablespoons olive oil

1 small onion, chopped

1 teaspoon ground cumin

3 cups low-salt chicken broth

2 (15-ounce) cans chickpeas, rinsed and drained

1 clove garlic, minced

6 cups baby spinach

½ cup shredded cotija cheese

Heat the oil in a soup pot over medium heat. Add the onion and cumin and sauté for 5 minutes until golden. Stir in the broth, chickpeas, and garlic. Bring the soup to a boil, then reduce the heat to medium-low and simmer for 15 minutes. Stir in baby spinach and cook for about 2 minutes, until the spinach has just wilted.

(continued)

Let cool slightly. When the soup is cool enough to handle, transfer half to a blender and puree until smooth. Return the puree to the pot and stir to combine.

Divide the soup among 4 soup bowls. Garnish each serving with 2 tablespoons of cheese.

PER SERVING: Protein: 2, Vegetables: 1, Healthy fats: ½

Quick Lentil Soup *Serves 4*

▶ (GRAIN DROP and CLEAN 16)

Save time by using canned lentils in this warm, comforting soup.

- 2 tablespoons olive oil
- 1 medium onion, chopped
- 1 cup chopped carrot
- 1 cup chopped celery
- 1 garlic clove, minced
- 1 teaspoon dried parsley
- 1 bay leaf
- 4 cups low-salt chicken or vegetable broth
- 1 (15-ounce) can crushed tomatoes
- 2 (15-ounce) cans lentils, rinsed and drained
- 1 tablespoon balsamic vinegar

Heat the oil in a soup pot over medium heat. Add the onion, carrot, celery, and garlic and sauté for 5 minutes, until the vegetables start to soften.

Add all the remaining ingredients. Bring the mixture just to a boil, then reduce the heat, cover, and simmer for 10 minutes. Discard the bay leaf.

Ladle into 4 soup bowls.

PER SERVING: Protein: 2, Vegetables: 2, Healthy fats: ½

Main Dishes

~~~~~~~

Seared Steak Chimichurri *Serves 4*

▶ (GRAIN DROP and CLEAN 16)

Garlicky, parsley-rich chimichurri sauce hails from Argentina and Uruguay and makes a fresh, sprightly topping for the grilled meat.

FOR THE CHIMICHURRI:

2 cloves garlic, peeled

1 cup packed fresh flat-leaf parsley

3 plum tomatoes, quartered

2 tablespoons fresh oregano leaves

3 tablespoons olive oil

1 tablespoon fresh lemon juice

½ teaspoon coarse salt

FOR THE STEAK:

1¼ pounds flank steak

3 teaspoons olive oil

1 teaspoon chili powder

4 medium ears corn, husked

To make the chimichurri, place the garlic in a food processor and process until finely minced. Add the parsley, tomatoes, oregano, the 3 tablespoons oil, the lemon juice, and salt and pulse until chunky.

To make the steak, preheat a grill to medium (or place an oven rack on the highest level and turn on the broiler). Coat the steak on both sides with 1 teaspoon of the oil and rub with the chili powder.

Place the steak on the grill (or on a foil-lined broiler pan) and cook for 5 minutes. Turn and cook for another 5 minutes for medium. Transfer the steak to a cutting board to rest for 10 minutes.

Brush the corn with the remaining 2 teaspoons oil and place the ears on the grill (or the same broiler pan) and cook for 3 minutes. Turn and cook for 3 minutes more.

When the steak has rested, cut across the grain into ½-inch-thick slices.

Lay out 4 plates and place an even portion of meat and an ear of corn on each one. Drizzle the meat and corn with chimichurri.

PER SERVING: Protein: 4, Vegetables: 3, Healthy fats: 1

Pork Tenderloin with Warm Salsa Verde *Serves 4*

▶ (GRAIN DROP and CLEAN 16)

Smoky green salsa verde has a fresh, tangy brightness from the tomatillos and cilantro. It also makes a tasty topping for broiled fish and chicken.

FOR THE SALSA VERDE:

- 2 cloves garlic, peeled
- ½ pound fresh tomatillos, husked and rinsed
- 2 scallions, trimmed
- 2 jalapeño peppers
- 2 tablespoons chopped fresh cilantro
- 2 tablespoons olive oil
- ½ cup low-salt chicken broth
- 1 tablespoon fresh lime juice

FOR THE PORK:

- 1¼ pounds pork tenderloin
- 2 tablespoons olive oil
- 8 cups baby spinach leaves

To make the salsa verde, place an oven rack on the highest level and turn on the broiler. Evenly scatter the garlic, tomatillos, scallions, and jalapeños on a foil-lined broiler pan. Broil the vegetables until blistered all over, turning often, and removing each one as it browns.

Stem and seed the jalapeños and add to a blender along with the garlic, tomatillos, scallions, and cilantro. Blend until pureed.

Heat the 2 tablespoons oil in a large skillet over medium heat. Add the pureed tomatillo mixture and cook for 5 minutes. Stir in the broth and bring the mixture to a boil. Reduce the heat to medium and simmer sauce until thickened, about 5 minutes. Stir in the lime juice.

To make the pork, preheat the broiler. Trim any visible fat from the tenderloin and slice off the silvery sheath. Place the pork on the same foil-lined broiler pan used to cook the vegetables and coat the meat with 1 tablespoon of the oil. Broil the pork for 10 minutes on each side. (Meat will be rosy but cooked through.) Transfer to a cutting board and tent with foil for 5 minutes to rest.

Heat the remaining 1 tablespoon oil in a large skillet over medium heat. Add the spinach and sauté just until wilted, about 2 minutes.

Lay out 4 dinner plates and place an even portion of spinach on each one. Cut the pork into thin slices and arrange even portions over the greens. Spoon the warm salsa verde over the pork.

PER SERVING: Protein: 4, Vegetables: 3, Healthy fats: 1

Mojito Salmon *Serves 4*

▶ (GRAIN DROP and CLEAN 16)

As with the mojito cocktail, lime and mint characterize the flavor of this sauce, enriched with avocado and crunchy jícama. This recipe is also delicious made with chicken, shrimp, or other types of fish.

FOR THE SALMON:

1 tablespoon olive oil

4 (5-ounce) pieces salmon, even thickness

FOR THE MOJITO TOPPING:

1½ cups diced cucumber

1½ cups diced peeled jícama

1 medium avocado, pitted, peeled, and diced

¼ cup chopped fresh mint

¼ cup fresh lime juice

1 tablespoon olive oil

¼ teaspoon salt

To make the salmon, heat the 1 tablespoon oil in a large nonstick skillet over medium heat. Place the fish, skin side down, in the skillet and cook for 6 minutes. Turn salmon and cook for 4 minutes more, or until just cooked through. Transfer the salmon to a plate and tent with foil.

To make the mojito topping, combine the cucumber, jícama, avocado, mint, lime juice, the 1 tablespoon oil, and the salt in a medium bowl. Stir to mix.

Lay out 4 plates. Peel the skin off the salmon (it should come off easily). Divide the fillets among the plates and smother with mojito topping.

PER SERVING: Protein: 4, Vegetables: 1, Healthy fats: 1½

Chicken Cutlets with Sherry Mushrooms *Serves 4*

▶ (GRAIN DROP and CLEAN 16)

Throughout Spain, you'll find crocks of sherry mushrooms in tapas bars. In this dish, these mushrooms make a flavorful topping for chicken cutlets. You'll notice that the recipe calls for a small amount of flour for dredging the chicken. Even when you're not eating any grains—as during the Grain Drop days—a little flour in a recipe like this is acceptable. If you'd prefer not to use wheat flour, you can opt for chickpea flour instead.

4 (5-ounce) boneless, skinless chicken breasts

1 egg white

¼ cup flour

3 tablespoons olive oil

2 cups sliced button mushrooms

1 cup sweet sherry

3 cloves garlic, minced

2 teaspoons minced fresh thyme

¼ teaspoon salt

4 cups baby spinach leaves

Place each chicken breast between two large pieces of plastic wrap and gently flatten with a meat mallet or the bottom of a heavy skillet until about ¼ inch thick.

Beat the egg white in a small bowl until frothy. Scatter the flour evenly on a large plate.

Heat 2 tablespoons of the oil in a large nonstick skillet over medium heat. Brush both sides of the cutlets with egg white and then dredge in flour. Shake off excess flour (discard any leftover flour). Place the cutlets in the pan and immediately turn each one to coat the other side with oil. Cook for 2 to 3 minutes per side, or until the cutlets are lightly browned and cooked through. Transfer to a plate and tent with foil to keep warm.

Add the remaining 1 tablespoon oil to the same skillet used to cook the chicken and heat over medium-high heat. Add the mushrooms and sauté until the mushrooms begin to brown, about 4 minutes. Stir in the sherry, garlic, thyme, and salt and simmer for 3 to 4 minutes, or until the sherry has reduced by half. Stir in the spinach and cook for about 1 minute, or until just wilted.

Lay out 4 plates. Place a chicken cutlet on each one and top with mushroom sauce.

PER SERVING: Protein: 4, Vegetables: 2, Healthy fats: 1

Brazilian Seafood Stew *Serves 4*

▶ (GRAIN DROP and CLEAN 16)

Clams give this stew a briny flavor, which plays off the sweetness of the coconut milk. Parsnip or winter squash chunks make a fine alternative to the plantain.

1 tablespoon olive oil

1 medium onion, chopped

2 cups chopped tomatoes

1 yellow bell pepper, chopped

2 cloves garlic, minced

1 teaspoon minced jalapeño pepper

1 (13.66-ounce) can light coconut milk

1 medium yellow plantain, peeled and cut into ½-inch-thick slices

8 hard-shell clams (littleneck or cherrystone)

1 cup water

1 pound skinless hake or cod, cut into chunks

½ pound medium shrimp, peeled and deveined

½ cup chopped fresh cilantro

Heat the oil in a soup pot over medium-low heat. Add the onion and sauté for about 3 minutes or until softened. Stir in the tomatoes, bell pepper, garlic, and jalapeño and cook for 2 minutes. Add the coconut milk and bring the mixture just to a boil. Add the plantain, reduce the heat to medium-low, and simmer, partially covered, for about 10 minutes, or until plantain is softened.

Add the clams and water. Cover and simmer for 5 to 6 minutes, or until the clams just open. Add the fish and shrimp and cook for 2 minutes more, until the seafood is just cooked through.

Lay out 4 large soup bowls. Spoon an even portion of stew into each bowl and garnish with cilantro.

PER SERVING: Protein: 6, Vegetables: 3, Healthy fats: 1

Smothered Flank Steak *Serves 4*

▶ (GRAIN DROP and CLEAN 16)

Letting meat rest after cooking allows it to reabsorb its juices, so when you cut the meat the juices stay in the steak rather than leaking out onto the cutting board.

2 tablespoons olive oil

1 large onion, sliced

1 large yellow bell pepper, cut into ¼-inch slices

1 large red bell pepper, cut into ¼-inch slices

2 cloves garlic, minced

1 chipotle pepper in adobo sauce, minced

1¼ pounds flank steak

1 teaspoon ground cumin

1 small avocado, pitted, peeled, and sliced

½ cup fat-free sour cream or Greek yogurt

½ cup chopped fresh cilantro

Heat 1 tablespoon of the oil in a large nonstick skillet over medium-high heat. Add the onion and bell peppers and sauté for about 10 minutes, or until the vegetables are soft. Stir in the garlic and chipotle. Transfer the mixture to a medium bowl and cover with foil to keep warm.

Rub the steak on both sides with the cumin. Add the remaining 1 tablespoon oil to the same skillet used to cook the vegetables and heat over medium-high heat. Add the steak and cook for 4 minutes on each side for medium. Transfer to a cutting board and tent with foil for 10 minutes to rest. When the steak has rested, cut across the grain into ½-inch-thick slices.

Lay out 4 plates. Place an equal amount of veggies on each plate and top with steak slices and avocado slices. Top each serving with 2 tablespoons each of sour cream and cilantro.

PER SERVING: Protein: 4, Vegetables: 1, Healthy fats: 1

Shrimp Veracruz over Cauliflower Rice *Serves 4*

▶ (GRAIN DROP and CLEAN 16)

Riced cauliflower is available in various stores, including Trader Joe's, which sells it frozen in bags. Or you can make your own by using a food processor or cheese grater to finely shred fresh cauliflower, omitting leaves and stem.

2 tablespoons olive oil	2 cloves garlic, minced
1 large onion, chopped	2 tablespoons capers, coarsely chopped
2 teaspoons minced jalapeño pepper	2 teaspoons minced fresh oregano
2 cups diced fresh tomatoes	1 (12-ounce) package riced cauliflower, fresh or frozen
½ cup seafood stock or low-salt chicken broth	1 ¼ pounds medium shrimp, peeled and deveined

Heat 1 tablespoon of the oil in a large sauté pan over medium heat. Add the onion and jalapeño and sauté for about 8 minutes, or until the onion is golden. Stir in the tomatoes, stock, garlic, capers, and oregano. Cook for 10 minutes. Reduce the heat to low.

Heat a medium nonstick skillet over medium-low heat. Add the remaining 1 tablespoon oil and the cauliflower, cover the skillet, and cook, stirring occasionally, for about 5 minutes or until the cauliflower rice is tender.

Add the shrimp to the tomato mixture and cook for 1 to 2 minutes, or until the shrimp is just cooked through.

Lay out 4 plates. Spoon an even portion of cauliflower rice onto each plate and top with shrimp mixture.

PER SERVING: Protein: 4, Vegetables: 3, Healthy fats: ½

Open-Face Pork Tacos with Spicy Pineapple Slaw *Serves 4*

▶ (CLEAN 16)

Restaurants throughout Mexico City serve open-face tacos, like these spicy pork tacos topped with a crunchy, sweet pineapple slaw.

FOR THE TACOS:

4 (6-inch) corn tortillas

1¼ pounds pork tenderloin

1 tablespoon olive oil

1 teaspoon ground coriander

1 teaspoon ground cumin

FOR THE PINEAPPLE SLAW:

2 cups thinly sliced cabbage

1 cup diced fresh pineapple

1 tablespoon olive oil

1 small avocado, pitted, peeled, and diced

1 serrano pepper, stemmed, seeded, and minced

¼ cup chopped fresh cilantro

2 scallions, thinly sliced

1 tablespoon fresh lime juice

To make the tacos, place a large skillet over medium-high heat. When hot, add one tortilla. Cook for 25 seconds per side or until blistered on each side. Continue with the remaining tortillas. Wrap in foil to keep warm.

Place an oven rack on the highest level and turn on the broiler. Trim any visible fat from the tenderloin and slice off the silvery sheath. Place the pork on a foil-lined broiler pan and coat with the 1 tablespoon oil. Blend the coriander and cumin in a small bowl and sprinkle over the pork. Broil the pork for 10 minutes on each side. (Meat will be rosy but cooked through.) Transfer to a cutting board and tent with foil for 5 minutes to rest before cutting into thin slices.

To make the pineapple slaw, place the cabbage and pineapple in a medium bowl and gently toss to mix. Add the 1 tablespoon oil, the avocado, serrano, cilantro, scallions, and lime juice. Gently toss again.

Lay out 4 plates. Place a corn tortilla on each plate and top with an even portion of slaw. Top the slaw with pork slices, and use a knife and fork to eat.

PER SERVING: Protein: 4, Vegetables: 1, Grains: 1, Healthy fats: 1

Brazilian Feijoada *Serves 4*

▶ (GRAIN DROP and CLEAN 16)

Low-fat turkey kielbasa replaces the fatty cuts of pork and beef normally used in this Latin dish. Sautéed collard greens, which we've added to the stew, often are served alongside.

2 tablespoons olive oil

1 medium onion, chopped

1 teaspoon dried thyme

1 cup low-salt chicken broth

2 cloves garlic, minced

2 cups chopped collard greens

½ pound smoked turkey kielbasa, sliced into coins

2 (15-ounce) cans black beans, rinsed and drained

Heat the oil in a large skillet over medium-high heat. Add the onion and thyme and sauté for 5 minutes, until the onion is golden. Add the broth, garlic, collards, kielbasa, and black beans. Simmer, partially covered, over low heat, stirring occasionally, for 45 minutes.

Divide the *feijoada* among 4 soup or pasta bowls.

PER SERVING: Protein: 4, Vegetables: 1, Healthy fats: ½

Loaded Shrimp Ceviche *Serves 4*

▶ (GRAIN DROP and CLEAN 16)

This makes a nice lunch, appetizer, or even cocktail nibble for a festive gathering.

1 pound cooked and peeled small shrimp

1 cup diced fresh tomatoes

1 cup diced cucumber

1 cup diced jícama

1 yellow bell pepper, diced

1 small serrano pepper, stemmed, seeded, and minced

1 medium avocado, pitted, peeled, and diced

½ cup cooked corn

¼ cup chopped red onion

¼ cup chopped fresh cilantro

Juice of 1 lime

¼ teaspoon salt

(continued)

Combine the shrimp, tomatoes, cucumber, jícama, bell pepper, serrano, avocado, corn, onion, and cilantro in a medium bowl.

Add the lime juice and salt and toss to mix.

Heap even portions of ceviche into 4 large goblets or bowls.

PER SERVING: Protein: 4, Vegetables: 2, Healthy fats: 1

Latin Beans and Quinoa with Poached Eggs *Serves 4*

▸ (CLEAN 16)

Quinoa contains a natural coating, called saponin, which if not rinsed off can give the grain a bitter, soapy taste.

2 tablespoons olive oil	1 teaspoon ground cumin
1 medium onion, chopped	2 (15-ounce) cans red kidney beans, rinsed and drained
1 green bell pepper, chopped	
1 red bell pepper, chopped	1 cup quinoa, rinsed in a fine-mesh sieve
1 jalapeño pepper, stemmed, halved lengthwise, and seeded	2 cloves garlic, minced
1 teaspoon dried thyme	4 eggs
1½ cups low-salt chicken broth	½ cup chopped fresh cilantro
1 teaspoon chili powder	1 cup salsa, fresh or from a jar

Heat the oil in a medium saucepan over medium heat. Add the onion, bell peppers, jalapeño, and thyme and cook for about 5 minutes, or until the vegetables begin to soften. Add the broth, chili powder, and cumin, scraping up any browned bits that have stuck to the bottom of the pot. Stir in the kidney beans, quinoa, and garlic. Bring to a boil, then reduce the heat to low, cover, and cook for 12 to 15 minutes, or until the broth is absorbed and the quinoa is tender. Fluff with a fork, cover, and let rest. If desired, discard the jalapeño halves.

Place a large skillet on the stove and fill one-third of the way with water. Bring the water to a boil, reduce the heat to medium, and crack and add the eggs one at a time. Poach the eggs for about 3 minutes, or until the center is still runny.

(continued)

Divide the quinoa among 4 shallow bowls. Top each with a poached egg and some cilantro. Serve salsa on the side.

PER SERVING: Protein: 3, Vegetables: 2, Grains: 1, Healthy fats: ½

Arroz con Pollo *Serves 4*

▶ (CLEAN 16)

This traditional dish has dozens of variations depending on who is making it and where it's made. This version uses brown rice, which adds fiber to the dish. Add a few shakes of hot sauce if you like a spicier taste.

- 2 tablespoons olive oil
- 1 medium onion, chopped
- 1 green bell pepper, chopped
- 1 cup low-salt chicken broth
- 1 (14.5-ounce) can diced tomatoes
- 2 cups cooked brown rice (⅓ cup uncooked)
- 1¼ pounds boneless, skinless chicken breasts, cut into chunks
- 3 cloves garlic, minced
- 6 whole pickled jalapeño peppers, minced
- 2 cups frozen baby peas

Heat the oil in a large skillet fitted with a lid over medium-high heat. Add the onion and bell pepper and sauté for 6 minutes, until the onion is golden. Stir in the broth, tomatoes, brown rice, chicken, garlic, and jalapeños. Bring the mixture just to a boil. Reduce the heat to medium-low, partially cover, and simmer for 10 minutes. Stir in the peas and cook for 5 minutes more to heat through. Let rest for 5 minutes.

Portion the chicken and rice mixture onto 4 plates.

PER SERVING: Protein: 4, Vegetables: 3, Grains: 1, Healthy fats: ½

Pork Fajitas with Salsa Crema *Serves 4*

▸ (CLEAN 16)

Pork tenderloin is so lean that when cut into strips, it cooks very quickly.

FOR THE SALSA CREMA:

1 single-serve container plain fat-free Greek yogurt

¼ cup prepared salsa

FOR THE FAJITAS:

4 (6-inch) whole grain corn or flour tortillas

1 ¼ pounds lean pork loin, cut into strips 2 inches long and ¼ inch thick

1 ½ teaspoons chili powder

1 teaspoon ground cumin

1 teaspoon garlic powder

2 tablespoons olive oil

1 red bell pepper, cut into strips

1 yellow bell pepper, cut into strips

1 large onion, sliced lengthwise

1 medium avocado, pitted, peeled, and sliced

To make the salsa crema, blend together the yogurt and salsa in a small bowl.

To make the fajitas, place a large nonstick skillet over medium-high heat. When hot, add a tortilla and cook for about 5 seconds per side until warm. Continue with the remaining tortillas. Wrap in foil to keep warm.

Place the pork strips in a medium bowl and toss with the chili powder, cumin, and garlic powder.

Heat the oil in the skillet over medium-high heat. Add the bell peppers and onion and cook for 6 minutes, until the vegetables soften. Add the pork and cook for 4 to 5 minutes, or until the pork is rosy and just cooked through.

Lay out 4 plates and place a tortilla on each plate. Place a portion of pork mixture over each tortilla, followed by some avocado slices, and salsa crema. Roll up the tortilla and enjoy.

PER SERVING: Protein: 4, Vegetables: 1, Grains: 1, Healthy fats: 1 ½

Latin Stuffed Peppers *Serves 4*

▶ (CLEAN 16)

Every family has its own recipe for stuffed peppers. Here we've swapped out some of the meat found in typical recipes for pinto beans.

- 2 tablespoons olive oil
- ½ cup chopped onion
- 1 pound ground turkey breast
- 2 cups salsa, fresh or from a jar
- ½ cup corn kernels, fresh or frozen (if frozen, no need to thaw)
- 1 cup canned pinto beans, rinsed and drained
- 1½ cups cooked brown rice (½ cup uncooked)
- 1 teaspoon chili powder
- 1 teaspoon ground cumin
- ¼ teaspoon salt
- 4 yellow bell peppers, halved lengthwise and seeds removed
- ½ cup shredded smoked cheddar cheese

Preheat the oven to 350°F.

Heat the oil in a large nonstick skillet over medium-high heat. Add the onion and ground turkey and sauté for about 10 minutes, or until turkey is cooked through. Remove from heat and stir in ¾ cup of the salsa, the corn, pinto beans, rice, chili powder, cumin, and salt.

Arrange the bell pepper halves in a 9 x 13-inch baking dish and fill the cupped area with the turkey mixture. Cover the dish with foil and bake for 1 hour. Remove the foil and sprinkle the cheese over the peppers. Return to the oven and bake for 10 minutes longer, or until the cheese has melted.

Place 2 pepper halves on each of 4 plates. Serve with the remaining 1¼ cups salsa, heated if desired.

PER SERVING: Protein: 4, Vegetables: 3, Grains: ½, Healthy fats: ½

Broiled Red Snapper with Fresh Mango Chutney *Serves 4*

▶ (GRAIN DROP and CLEAN 16)

This is a very versatile recipe in that you can use any ripe, juicy fruit in place of mango (pineapple, papaya, etc.) and chicken or even pork tenderloin instead of the fish.

FOR THE CHUTNEY:

- 1 large mango
- 1 red bell pepper, chopped
- 1 teaspoon minced jalapeño pepper
- ¼ cup chopped fresh cilantro
- Juice of 1 lime
- ¼ teaspoon ground cumin

FOR THE SNAPPER:

- 1¼ pounds red snapper or other white fish fillets
- 2 teaspoons olive oil
- ½ teaspoon garlic powder
- ¼ teaspoon salt

To make the chutney, slice the mango lengthwise along either side of the pit so that you have three pieces: two halves and a central section holding the pit. For each of the halves, use a sharp knife to cut through the flesh (without going through the skin) in a crosshatch pattern. Using a spoon, scoop the mango cubes from the skin into a small bowl. Cut the skin off the remaining central section and cut the fruit around the pit into small chunks. Add to the bowl. Add the bell pepper, jalapeño, cilantro, lime juice, and cumin. Toss the mixture gently to combine.

To make the fish, place an oven rack on the highest level and turn on the broiler. Place the snapper, skin side down, on a foil-lined broiler pan. Brush the fish with the oil and sprinkle with the garlic powder and salt. Broil for 10 to 12 minutes, or until the fish flakes easily. Slide a spatula under fish—the skin should stick to the foil.

Divide the fish among 4 plates and top with fresh mango chutney.

PER SERVING: Protein: 4, Vegetables: 1

Spanish Tomato Toasts *Serves 4*

▶ (CLEAN 16)

Plain tomato toast is served in cafés all over Spain, particularly for the first meal of the day. Here, we've added protein with white beans and Spanish cheese.

12 slices (½-inch thick) from a whole wheat baguette (save the remaining bread for another use)

2 tablespoons olive oil

2 medium tomatoes, each halved horizontally

2 cloves garlic, halved

1 (15-ounce) can white beans, rinsed and drained

4 ounces Manchego cheese, grated

Preheat the oven to 400°F.

Place the bread slices on a baking sheet. Brush both sides of each slice with the oil. Bake for about 8 minutes, or until the bread is crispy and lightly browned.

Meanwhile, using a box grater, grate each tomato half into a large bowl, discarding the core and skin. Transfer the tomato pulp to a fine-mesh sieve to drain.

When the bread is toasted, rub the cut garlic around the crust of each bread slice. Place 3 toasts on each of 4 plates. Spoon an even portion of tomato pulp over each toast, and top with beans and cheese.

PER SERVING: Protein: 2, Vegetables: 1, Grains: 1, Healthy fats: ½

Garlicky Lime Shrimp *Serves 4*

▶ (GRAIN DROP and CLEAN 16)

Garlic, lime, and shrimp combine to make a quick, delicious dish that is fabulous over pureed butternut squash, cauliflower rice, or quinoa.

2 tablespoons olive oil

1 medium onion, chopped

1 ¼ pounds large shrimp, peeled and deveined

6 cloves garlic, minced

8 cups baby spinach leaves

¼ teaspoon salt

¼ teaspoon red pepper flakes

1 tablespoon fresh lime juice

¼ cup chopped fresh cilantro

Heat the oil in a large skillet over medium-high heat. Add the onion and sauté for 5 minutes until golden. Add the shrimp, garlic, spinach, salt, and red pepper flakes and cook for 2 to 3 minutes, or until the shrimp is just cooked through. Remove from the heat and stir in the lime juice.

Divide the shrimp mixture among 4 plates and sprinkle with cilantro.

PER SERVING: Protein: 4, Vegetables: 2, Healthy fats: ½

Catalan Fish Stew *Serves 4*

▶ (GRAIN DROP and CLEAN 16)

Saffron and almonds give this stew richness and depth, while the sweetness in the sherry balances the brininess of the seafood.

2 tablespoons olive oil

1 medium onion, chopped

1 medium tomato, diced

Pinch of saffron threads

3 cups low-salt chicken broth or fish stock

¼ cup cream sherry

1 pound waxy potatoes, quartered and sliced

12 small clams (Manila, littleneck, or cherrystone)

10 almonds, skin on

2 cloves garlic, peeled

¼ cup chopped fresh parsley

½ pound skinless firm white fish fillets (such as hake, cod, or halibut), cut into chunks

½ pound medium shrimp, peeled and deveined

(continued)

Heat the oil in a soup pot over medium heat. Add the onion and sauté for 5 minutes, until golden. Stir in the tomato and saffron and sauté for 5 minutes more to break down the saffron.

Add the broth, sherry, and potatoes. Bring the mixture just to a boil, then reduce the heat to medium-low and simmer for 15 minutes. Add the clams, cover the pot, and simmer for 10 minutes more, or until the clams just open.

Place the almonds, garlic, and parsley in a food processor and process until ground. Stir the mixture into the stew, along with the fish and shrimp. Cook for 1 to 2 minutes, or until the seafood is just cooked through.

Ladle the stew into 4 large soup or pasta bowls.

PER SERVING: Protein: 4, Vegetables: 3, Nuts/seeds: 0 (amount is so small that we'll call it 0), Healthy fats: ½

Spicy Cheese and Refried Bean Quesadillas *Serves 4*

▶ (CLEAN 16)

Whole grain tortillas add fiber to these cheesy, beany bites.

1 (16-ounce) can vegetarian refried beans

2 teaspoons ground cumin

1 teaspoon hot sauce

4 (12-inch) whole grain flour tortillas

1 (6-ounce) jar sliced roasted red peppers, drained

1 cup shredded Jack cheese

1 cup salsa, fresh or from a jar

Stir together the refried beans, cumin, and hot sauce in a small bowl.

Spread each tortilla with one-quarter of the bean mixture. Arrange some red peppers over one-half of the refried beans. Sprinkle cheese over the peppers. Fold each tortilla in half to create a half-moon shape.

Place a large nonstick skillet over medium heat. Working in batches, cook 2 quesadillas for 2 to 3 minutes on each side, or until lightly browned.

Serve each quesadilla on a plate with some salsa.

PER SERVING: Protein: 2, Grains: 2

Chicken Cutlets with Veggie Pico de Gallo *Serves 4*

▶ (GRAIN DROP and CLEAN 16)

Although pico de gallo is similar to salsa, it typically contains less liquid. This version is packed with vegetables and avocado.

1 cup chopped fresh tomatoes

½ cup corn kernels, fresh or frozen (thawed if frozen)

½ cup chopped jícama

½ cup chopped zucchini

½ cup chopped fresh cilantro

¼ cup minced onion

1 small avocado, pitted, peeled, and diced

1 tablespoon fresh lime juice

¼ teaspoon salt

2 tablespoons olive oil

4 (5-ounce) boneless, skinless chicken breasts (1¼ pounds total)

1 egg white

¼ cup flour

Combine the tomatoes, corn, jícama, zucchini, cilantro, onion, avocado, lime juice, salt, and 1 tablespoon of the oil in a small bowl. Toss to mix.

Place each chicken breast between two large pieces of plastic wrap and gently flatten with a meat mallet or the bottom of a heavy skillet until ¼ inch thick.

Place the egg white in a small bowl and beat until frothy. Scatter the flour evenly on a large plate.

Brush both sides of the cutlets with egg white and dredge in flour. Shake off excess flour (discard any unused flour). Heat the remaining 1 tablespoon oil in a large nonstick skillet over medium heat. Place the cutlets in the pan and immediately turn to coat the other side with oil. Cook for 2 to 3 minutes per side, or until the cutlet is lightly browned and cooked through.

Lay out 4 plates. Place a cutlet on each plate and top with an even portion of pico de gallo mixture.

PER SERVING: Protein: 4, Vegetables: 1, Healthy fats: 1

Veggie Burrito Bowl *Serves 4*

▶ (GRAIN DROP and CLEAN 16)

Easy to assemble, fresh, and delicious. This veggie dish also packs nicely for a healthy lunch to go.

2 tablespoons olive oil

2 ½ tablespoons fresh lime juice

1 clove garlic, minced

¼ teaspoon ground cumin

8 cups shredded romaine lettuce

2 cups canned black beans, rinsed and drained

2 cups corn kernels, fresh or frozen (thawed if frozen)

1 small avocado, pitted, peeled, and diced

1 red bell pepper, chopped

½ cup salsa, spicy or regular, fresh or from a jar

¾ cup shredded Monterey Jack cheese

Whisk together the oil, lime juice, garlic, and cumin in a small bowl. Set aside.

Lay out 4 large bowls. In each bowl, place 2 cups romaine lettuce followed by ½ cup black beans, ½ cup corn, one-quarter of the avocado, one-quarter of the bell pepper, 2 tablespoons salsa, and one-quarter of the cheese.

Drizzle an even portion of dressing over each serving.

PER SERVING: Protein: 2, Vegetables: 3, Healthy fats: 1

Spicy Fish Tacos with Cool Avocado Slaw *Serves 4*

▶ (CLEAN 16)

These tacos come together in a flash. They're also good with shrimp and chicken. Serve with your favorite hot sauce.

FOR THE SLAW:

- 1 medium avocado, pitted and peeled
- 1 single-serve container plain fat-free Greek yogurt
- 1 tablespoon fresh lime juice
- ¼ cup chopped fresh cilantro
- ¼ teaspoon salt
- 2 cups thinly sliced red cabbage

FOR THE TACOS:

- 8 (6-inch) corn tortillas
- 1 teaspoon chili powder
- 1 teaspoon garlic powder
- 1¼ pounds skinless salmon or firm white fish (halibut or cod) fillets
- 1 tablespoon olive oil

To make the slaw, mash the avocado in a medium bowl. Blend in the yogurt, lime juice, cilantro, and salt. Add the cabbage and toss to coat with the dressing.

To make the tacos, place a large nonstick skillet over medium-high heat. When hot, add a tortilla and cook for about 25 seconds per side or until blistered. Continue with the remaining tortillas. Wrap in foil to keep warm.

Blend the chili powder and garlic powder in a small bowl. Coat the fish with the spice mixture.

Heat the oil in a large nonstick skillet over medium-high heat. Add the fish and cook for 5 minutes. Flip and cook for 4 minutes more, or until the fish is just cooked through. Transfer the fillet to a plate. Cut into 8 pieces.

Arrange 2 tortillas on each of 4 plates and top each with even portions of slaw and fish.

PER SERVING: Protein: 4, Vegetables: 1, Grains: 2, Healthy fats: 1½

Pork Tenderloin with Black Bean Mojo *Serves 4*

▶ (GRAIN DROP and CLEAN 16)

Mojo is the term for a variety of spicy sauces that are made in such countries as Cuba, Spain, and Portugal. This one combines black beans and orange for a tasty topping for pork.

FOR THE MOJO:

1 tablespoon olive oil

2 cloves garlic, minced

¼ teaspoon ground cumin

¼ teaspoon dried oregano

1 tablespoon fresh lime juice

1 (15-ounce) can black beans, rinsed and drained

1 orange, peeled, separated into sections, and cut into bite-size pieces

2 tablespoons chopped fresh cilantro

FOR THE PORK:

1¼ pounds pork tenderloin

1 tablespoon olive oil

To make the mojo, heat 1 tablespoon oil in a small nonstick skillet over medium-low heat. Add the garlic, cumin, and oregano and gently sauté for 1 minute. Remove from heat and stir in the lime juice.

Place the black beans, orange, and cilantro in a bowl and stir in the garlic mixture.

To make the pork, place an oven rack on the highest level and turn on the broiler. Trim any visible fat from the tenderloin and slice off the silvery sheath. Place the pork on a foil-lined broiler pan and coat the meat with the 1 tablespoon oil. Broil the pork for 10 minutes on each side. (Meat will be rosy but cooked through.) Transfer to a cutting board and tent with foil for 5 minutes to rest.

Cut the pork into thin slices and divide among 4 plates. Spoon the black bean mojo over each serving.

PER SERVING: Protein: 5, Healthy fats: ½

Overstuffed Avocados *Serves 4*

▶ (GRAIN DROP and CLEAN 16)

Rich, buttery avocados hold a bright, crisp blend of healthy vegetables. The cheese adds a welcome savory note and the seeds add crunch.

1 cup corn kernels, fresh or frozen (thawed if frozen)

1 (14-ounce) can hearts of palm, drained and sliced

1 red bell pepper, diced

¼ cup chopped fresh cilantro

2 tablespoons olive oil

1 tablespoon fresh lime juice

½ cup salsa, fresh or from a jar

8 cups chopped romaine lettuce

2 medium avocados, pitted and peeled

¼ cup crumbled Queso Fresco cheese

¼ cup toasted hulled pumpkin seeds

Combine the corn, hearts of palm, bell pepper, cilantro, oil, lime juice, and salsa in a medium bowl. Gently stir to combine.

Spread 2 cups romaine on each of 4 plates. Nestle an avocado half, pitted-side up, on each bed of greens. Fill each avocado half with an even portion of corn mixture. Top each with 1 tablespoon Queso Fresco and pumpkin seeds.

PER SERVING: Protein: 0 (amount is so small that we'll call it 0), Vegetables: 3, Nuts/seeds: ½, Healthy fats: 2

Chile-Turkey Burgers with Mushroom Cap "Buns" *Serves 4*

▶ (GRAIN DROP and CLEAN 16)

Yes, it's a bit surprising to create burger buns from mushrooms, but it works and makes a delicious, grain-free substitute for the flour-based buns.

1 ¼ pounds ground turkey breast

½ cup diced onion

2 tablespoons canned green chilies, drained

1 teaspoon ground cumin

½ teaspoon salt

8 bun-size portobello mushroom caps, stems removed

2 tablespoons olive oil

4 (1-ounce) slices Jack cheese

4 tomato slices

Hot sauce, for serving

Combine the ground turkey, onion, chilies, cumin, and salt in a medium bowl and mix well. Divide the mixture into 4 equal portions and shape into patties about the diameter of the mushroom caps.

Heat a large nonstick skillet over medium-high heat. Brush the mushroom caps with 1 tablespoon of the oil and place in the skillet. Cook for 6 minutes, flip, and cook for another 6 minutes, or until the caps are juicy and cooked through. Transfer the caps to a platter.

Add the remaining 1 tablespoon oil to the same skillet used to cook the mushrooms and heat over medium heat. Add the patties, cook for 5 minutes, flip, and cook for 2 minutes more.

Place a slice of cheese on each patty. Cover the skillet, reduce the heat to low, and cook the burgers for 1 to 2 minutes more, or until cooked through and the cheese is melted.

Lay out 4 plates. Place a portobello "bun" stem side up on each plate, and top with a burger. Top each burger with a tomato slice and a mushroom "bun" top. Serve with hot sauce and plenty of napkins.

PER SERVING: Protein: 5, Vegetables: 1

Neo-Cuban Sandwich *Serves 4*

▶ (CLEAN 16)

We've pumped up this traditional favorite with healthy, filling veggies.

2 tablespoons olive oil

1 large onion, halved and thinly sliced

8 slices whole grain bread

Cooking spray

8 teaspoons prepared mustard

8 slices (1 ounce each) plain cooked turkey breast (from the deli section)

4 slices (1 ounce each) Swiss cheese

8 dill pickle sandwich slices, chopped

1 cup chopped watercress or baby spinach

8 tomato slices

Heat 1 tablespoon of the oil in a small nonstick skillet over medium-high heat. Add the onion and sauté for about 8 minutes, or until golden.

Lay out the bread slices and coat one side with cooking spray. Flip the slices over and spread each with 1 teaspoon mustard.

On each of 4 slices of bread, make these layers: 2 turkey slices, 1 cheese slice, even portions of cooked onion and pickle, ¼ cup watercress, and 2 tomato slices. Place the remaining 4 slices of bread mustard side down on top.

Heat the remaining 1 tablespoon oil in a large nonstick skillet over medium heat. Place the sandwiches in the pan. Place another heavy skillet on top of the sandwiches and cook for 4 minutes. Remove the top skillet, flip the sandwiches, and repeat the process on the second side, cooking for another 4 minutes.

Cut each sandwich in half and serve.

PER SERVING: Protein: 3, Vegetables: 1, Grains: 2, Healthy fats: ½

Baked Enchiladas with Roasted Vegetables *Serves 4*

▶ (CLEAN 16)

These require a bit of assembly, but once they're in the oven, your work is done. They reheat nicely and are also tasty cold.

Cooking spray

1 pound sweet potatoes, unpeeled, diced

2 red bell peppers, cut into thin wedges

1 large red onion, cut into thin wedges

1 tablespoon olive oil

1 teaspoon ground coriander

1 teaspoon ground cumin

½ teaspoon salt

3 cloves garlic, minced

8 (6-inch) corn tortillas

1½ cups shredded Pepper Jack cheese

4 cups prepared salsa, regular or spicy, fresh or from a jar

Preheat the oven to 400°F. Coat a large roasting pan and a 9 x 13-inch baking dish with cooking spray.

Combine the sweet potatoes, bell peppers, and onion in a medium bowl. Add the oil, coriander, cumin, and salt and toss to coat. Transfer the vegetables to the prepared roasting pan and bake for 40 minutes, turning occasionally, or until the vegetables are soft and golden.

Remove the vegetables from the oven and stir in the garlic. Leave the oven on but reduce the temperature to 350°F.

Place a medium nonstick skillet over medium heat. Add a tortilla and cook for 8 to 10 seconds on each side, or until the tortilla becomes soft and warm.

Place a tortilla on a flat surface and spoon one-eighth of the vegetable mixture down the center in a strip. Top with 2 tablespoons cheese. Roll up the tortilla and place, seam side down, in the prepared baking dish. Repeat to make a total of 8 enchiladas. Pour 2 cups of the salsa over the enchiladas. Bake for 20 minutes.

Sprinkle with the remaining ½ cup cheese and bake for 5 minutes more.

Place 2 enchiladas on each of 4 plates and serve with the remaining 2 cups salsa, warmed if desired.

PER SERVING: Protein: 1½, Vegetables: 4½, Grains: 2, Healthy fats: ½

South American Chicken and Squash Stew *Serves 4*

▶ (GRAIN DROP and CLEAN 16)

The chipotle pepper in adobo sauce, smoked paprika, and smoked kielbasa add a spicy richness to this chicken stew.

2 tablespoons olive oil

1 large onion, diced

½ pound smoked turkey kielbasa, cut into ½-inch-thick coins

¾ pounds boneless, skinless chicken breast, chopped

2 cups low-salt chicken broth

2 cups diced peeled butternut squash

2 medium carrots, peeled and sliced

2 cups frozen baby lima beans

1 chipotle pepper in adobo sauce, minced

1 teaspoon smoked paprika

Heat the oil in a Dutch oven (or other heavy cooking pot with a lid) over medium-high heat. Add the onion and kielbasa and sauté for 5 minutes, until the onion is golden. Add the chicken and sauté for 2 minutes.

Stir in the broth and scrape up any browned bits that have stuck to the bottom of the pot.

Add the squash, carrots, lima beans, chipotle, and smoked paprika. Bring the mixture to a boil, then reduce the heat to low and simmer the stew, partially covered, for 45 minutes.

Let the stew cool slightly before dividing among 4 shallow bowls.

PER SERVING: Protein: 5, Vegetables: 2, Healthy fats: ½

ACKNOWLEDGMENTS

Many people have contributed to the creation of this book, and I would like to offer my sincere thanks for their support.

My greatest appreciation goes to my family, especially my wife, Ana Raquel, and my children, Ana Sofia, Juan Antonio, and Nina. Everything I do, I do for them.

I am forever grateful to my mother, Carmen, and my father, Juan Manuel, who instilled in me a humble ambition that has no limits, no biases, and no frontiers, and whose main purpose and drive is to positively change the lives of others.

We all live through some very difficult professional times and cross-roads. I am no exception. There are angels in our lives who in one way or another help us push forward. In my case, that angel was Mr. José Rial. He opened an important door for me.

I'd also like to thank my patients and the fans of my television shows. It is an honor and a joy to help so many people, and to share their lives and their stories. When they stop me at an airport, shopping mall, or restaurant to ask my medical opinion on a problem they have, they make me fall in love with my profession even more.

I would not be where I am today without my mentors. Dr. Richard Lange's love for the practice of medicine is unparalleled, and I was infected by it. Dr. Roger Blumenthal introduced me to the wonderful world of cardiovascular prevention. Unselfish, enthusiastic, and extremely supportive, Roger is the quintessential mentor. These two gentlemen are my professional role models and, lucky for me, also my friends.

I am thankful to my clinic staff, Vanessa, Sonia, and Deny. Your efficiency and dedication allow me to do many things at once. I am also grateful to my big Univision family who have trusted and supported me for many years in order for me to deliver to our audience the information and tools they need to improve their lives.

Creating a book is a team effort, and I'd like to recognize all of the people who helped me bring this book to life.

Many thanks to Alice Lesch Kelly, who is much more than a writing partner. Alice is a sounding board and an accomplice during the idea-generating process. We came up with the name of this book during a brainstorming phone conversation; I can't remember the exact day, but judging by the title it must have been a Friday afternoon.

Thanks also to recipe developer Victoria Abbott Riccardi, whose extensive culinary skills and knowledge of world cuisines guided her to create a fantastic collection of delicious, healthy recipes.

And finally, a big thank-you to the team at Atria Books, especially my editors, Johanna Castillo and Sarah Pelz, who believed in my vision for creating a weight-loss plan that is built around celebration and joy, and assistant editor Melanie Iglesias, who sweated all the details.

RESOURCES

Agricultural Research Service, United States Department of Agriculture, https://www.ars.usda.gov/

American Academy of Family Physicians, https://familydoctor.org/

American Cancer Society, https://www.cancer.org/

American Council on Exercise, https://www.acefitness.org/

American Diabetes Association, http://www.diabetes.org/

American Heart Association, https://www.heart.org/

American Lamb Board, http://www.americanlamb.com/

Centers for Disease Control and Prevention, https://www.cdc.gov/

Choose My Plate, United States Department of Agriculture, https://www.choosemyplate.gov/

Common Health, WBUR, http://commonhealth.legacy.wbur.org/

Harvard Medical School, https://www.health.harvard.edu/

Healthy for GoodTM, American Heart Association, https://healthyforgood.heart.org/

Johns Hopkins Medicine, Colorectal Cancer Center, https://www.hopkinsmedicine.org/kimmel_cancer_center/centers/colorectal_cancer/index.html

Mayo Clinic, https://www.mayoclinic.org/

MedlinePlus (US National Library of Medicine), https://medlineplus.gov/

National Academies of Sciences, Engineering, and Medicine, http://www.nationalacademies.org/

National Cancer Institute, https://www.cancer.gov/

National Center for Complementary and Integrative Health, https://nccih.nih.gov/

National Heart, Lung, and Blood Institute, https://www.nhlbi.nih.gov/

National Institute of Diabetes and Digestive and Kidney Diseases, https://www.niddk.nih.gov/

National Institute on Alcohol Abuse and Alcoholism, https://www.niaaa.nih.gov/

National Pork Board, https://www.pork.org/

Nutrition Source, Harvard School of Public Health, https://www.hsph.harvard.edu/nutritionsource/

Office of Dietary Supplements, https://ods.od.nih.gov/

Office of Disease Prevention and Health Promotion, https://health.gov/

Truvia FAQ: Health Information and Safety, https://www.truvia.com/faq#faq_1

United States Food and Drug Administration, https://www.fda.gov/

Articles

Abargouei, A. S. et al. "Effect of Dairy Consumption on Weight and Body Composition in Adults: A Systematic Review and Meta-Analysis of Randomized Controlled Clinical Trials." *International Journal of Obesity* 36 (2012): 1485–93. https://www.ncbi.nlm.nih.gov/pubmed/22249225

Abdel-Aal, E.-S. "Dietary Sources of Lutein and Zeaxanthin Carotenoids and Their Role in Eye Health." *Nutrients* 5, no. 4 (April 2013): 1169–85. https://www.ncbi.nlm.nih.gov/pmc /articles /PMC3705341/

Alexander, D. D. et al. "Meta-analysis of Egg Consumption and Risk of Coronary Heart Disease and Stroke." *Journal of the American College of Nutrition* (October 6, 2016): 1–13. https://www.ncbi.nlm.nih.gov/pubmed /27710205

Azad, M. B. et al. "Nonnutritive Sweeteners and Cardiometabolic Health: A Systematic Review and Meta-Analysis of Randomized Controlled Trials and Prospective Cohort Studies." *CMAJ* 189, no. 28 (July 17, 2017): E929–E939. http://www.cmaj.ca/content/189/28/E929

Bell, Steven et al. "Association Between Clinically Recorded Alcohol Consumption and Initial Presentation of 12 Cardiovascular Diseases: Population Based Cohort Study Using Linked Health Records." *BMJ* (2017); 356: j909. http://www.bmj.com/content/bmj/356/bmj.j909.full.pdf

Blom, W. et al. "Effect of a High-Protein Breakfast on the Postprandial Ghrelin Response." *American Journal of Clinical Nutrition* 83, no. 2 (February 2006): 211–20. http://ajcn.nutrition .org/content/83/2/211 .abstract?ijkey=82c915361bb4a86d3c7c5e440099640c69ce5975&key type2=tf_ipsecsha

Blumenthal, J. A. "Effects of the DASH Diet Alone and in Combination with Exercise and Weight Loss on Blood Pressure and Cardiovascular Biomarkers in Men and Women with High Blood Pressure." *Archives of Internal Medicine* 170, no. 2 (2010): 126–35. https://jamanetwork .com /journals/jamainternalmedicine/fullarticle/415515

Carlsen, M. H. et al. "The Total Antioxidant Content of More than 3,100 Foods, Beverages, Spices, Herbs, and Supplements Used Worldwide." *Nutrition Journal* (January 22, 2010); 9:3. https://www.ncbi.nlm.nih .gov/pubmed /20096093

Collier, R. "Intermittent Fasting: The Science of Going Without." *CMAJ* 185, no. 9 (June 11, 2013); E363–64. https://www.ncbi.nlm.nih.gov /pmc/articles/PMC3680567/

Daley, C. A. "A Review of Fatty Acid Profiles and Antioxidant Content in Grass-Fed and Grain-Fed Beef." *Nutrition Journal* 10, no. 9 (March 2010): 10. https://nutritionj.biomedcentral.com /articles/10.1186 /1475-2891-9-10

DiMarco, D. M. et al. "Intake of up to 3 Eggs per Day Is Associated with Changes in HDL Function and Increased Plasma Antioxidants in Healthy, Young Adults." *Journal of Nutrition* (January 11, 2017): 241877. http://jn.nutrition.org/content/early/2017/01/10/jn .116.241877

Etemadi, A. et al. "Mortality from Different Causes Associated with Meat, Heme Iron, Nitrates, and Nitrites in the NIH-AARP Diet and Health Study: Population-Based Cohort Study." *BMJ* (2017): 357; j1957. http://www.bmj.com/content/357/bmj.j1957

Guasch-Ferré, M. et al. "Nut Consumption and Risk of Cardio-vascular Disease." *Journal of the American College of Cardiology* 70, no. 20 (November 2017). http://www.onlinejacc.org /content/70/20/2519?sso=1&sso_redirect_count=5&access_token=

Izadi, V. "Dietary Intakes and Leptin Concentrations." *ARYA Atherosclerosis* 10, no. 5 (September 2014): 266–72. https://www.ncbi.nlm.nih.gov/pmc/articles/PMC4251481/

Jannasch, F. "Dietary Patterns and Type 2 Diabetes: A Systematic Literature Review and Meta-Analysis of Prospective Studies." *Journal of Nutrition* 147, no. 6 (June 2017): 1174–82. http://jn.nutrition.org/content/early/2017/04/19/jn.116.242552.abstract

"Keeping a Food Diary Doubles Weight Loss, Study Suggests." Kaiser Permanente press release. https://www.sciencedaily.com/releases/2008/07/080708080738.htm

Leidy, H. J. et al. "The Role of Protein in Weight Loss and Maintenance." *American Journal of Clinical Nutrition* 101, no. 6 (June 2015): 1320S–1329S. http://ajcn.nutrition.org/content/101/6/1320S.long

Longland, T. M. et al. "Higher Compared with Lower Dietary Protein during an Energy Deficit Combined with Intense Exercise Promotes Greater Lean Mass Gain and Fat Mass Loss: A Randomized Clinical Trial." *American Journal of Clinical Nutrition* 103, no. 3 (March 2016): 738–46. http://ajcn.nutrition.org/content/103/3/738

Ma, Y. et al. "Single Component vs. Multicomponent Dietary Goals for the Metabolic Syndrome: A Randomized Trial." *Annals of Internal Medicine* 162, no. 4 (2015): 248–57. http:// annals.org/aim/article-abstract/2118594/single-component-versus-multicomponent-dietary-goals-metabolic-syndrome-randomized-trial

Mattson, M. P., and R. Wan. "Beneficial Effects of Intermittent Fasting and Caloric Restriction on the Cardiovascular and Cerebrovascular System." *Journal of Nutritional Biochemistry* 16, no. 3 (March 2005): 129–37. http://www.sciencedirect.com/science/article/pii/S095528630400261X ?via%3Dihub

Mayor, S. "Diet High in Vegetables, Fruit, and Whole Grains May Reduce Risk of Gout." *BMJ* (2017); j2238. http://www.bmj.com/content/357/bmj.j2238

Moore, S. C. et al. "Leisure Time Physical Activity of Moderate to Vigorous Intensity and Mortality: A Large Pooled Cohort Analysis." *PLOS*

Medicine 9, no. 11 (2012): e1001335. http://journals.plos.org/plos medicine/article?id=10.1371/journal.pmed.1001335

Morris, M. C. "MIND Diet Associated with Reduced Incidence of Alzheimer's Disease." *Alzheimer's and Dementia* 11, no. 9 (September 2015): 1007–14. http://www .alzheimersanddementia.com/article /S1552-5260%2815%2900017-5/abstract

"New MIND Diet May Significantly Protect Against Alzheimer's Disease." Rush University Medical Center. https://www.rush.edu/news/press -releases/new-mind-diet-may-significantly-protect-against-alzheimers -disease

Nichols, G. A. "Cardiometabolic Risk Factors among 1.3 Million Adults with Overweight or Obesity, but Not Diabetes, in 10 Geographically Diverse Regions of the United States, 2012–2013." *Preventing Chronic Disease* 14: 160438 (2017). https://www.cdc.gov/pcd /issues /2017 /16_0438.htm#table2_down

Pan, A. et al. "Red Meat Consumption and Mortality: Results from 2 Prospective Cohort Studies." *Archives of Internal Medicine* 172, no. 7 (2012): 555–63. https://jamanetwork.com /journals/jamainternalmedicine /fullarticle/1134845

"Sleep Deprivation Linked to Junk Food Cravings." *UC Berkeley News*. http://news.berkeley.edu/2013/08/06/poor-sleep-junk-food/

Sotos-Prieto, M. et al. "Association of Changes in Diet Quality with Total and Cause-Specific Mortality." *New England Journal of Medicine* (2017); 377: 143–53. http://www.nejm.org/doi/full /10.1056 /NEJMoa1613502

Steven, S. et al. "Very Low-Calorie Diet and 6 Months of Weight Stability in Type 2 Diabetes: Pathophysiological Changes in Responders and Nonresponders." *Diabetes Care* 39, no. 5 (May 2016): 808–15. http:// care.diabetesjournals.org/content/39/5/88

Van Elswyk, M. E., and S. H. McNeill. "Impact of Grass/Forage Feeding vs. Grain Finishing on Beef Nutrients and Sensory Quality: The US Experience." *Meat Science* 96, no. 1 (January 2014): 535–40. https:// www.sciencedirect.com/science/article/pii/S0309174013004944

Wei, M. et al. "Fasting Mimicking Diet and Markers/Risk Factors for

Aging, Diabetes, Cancer, and Cardiovascular Disease." *Science Translational Medicine* 9, no. 377 (15 Feb 2017) eaai8700. http://stm .sciencemag.org/content/9/377/eaai8700

Westerterp, K. R. "Diet Induced Thermogenesis." *Nutrition and Metabolism* 1, no. 5 (2004). https://www.ncbi.nlm.nih.gov/pmc/articles /PMC524030/

"Zumba Dance Improves Health in Overweight/Obese Type 2 Diabetic Women." *American Journal of Health Behavior* 39, no. 1 (January 2015): 109–120 (12). http://www.ingentaconnect .com/content/png /ajhb/2015/00000039/00000001/art00012

"58% Eat at a Restaurant at Least Once a Week." *Rasmussen Reports*. http:// www.rasmussenreports.com/public_content/lifestyle/general_lifestyle /july_2013/58_eat_at_a_restaurant_at_least_once_a_week

INDEX

ABOUT THE AUTHOR

Juan Rivera, MD, is a board-certified cardiologist and internist who trained at The Johns Hopkins Hospital. He specializes in the prevention, early detection, and treatment of cardiovascular diseases, and empowers people by providing them with the tools and knowledge they need to prevent illness.

Dr. Juan serves as the chief medical correspondent for the Univision TV network and hosts his own wildly popular one-hour program on Univision, *Dr. Juan*. He has published extensively in the area of cardiovascular disease prevention and serves as a reviewer for most major peer-reviewed scientific cardiology journals. He speaks to audiences around the world about cardiovascular disease prevention.

A native of San Juan, Puerto Rico, Dr. Juan practices cardiology in Miami Beach, Florida, where he has a successful concierge cardiology practice.